S T R E T C H E D

Build Your Yoga Business, Grow Your Teaching Techniques

by Karen Fabian

Nicole,
*   Keep on*
*   stretching!*
thanks for being a
good friend!
*   xo*
*   Khn*

ISBN-13: 978-1499701142
ISBN-10: 1499701144

Book Website
www.barebonesyoga.com
Email: karen@barebonesyoga.com.

Printed in U.S.A

I'd like to dedicate this book to the greatest teachers I've ever had: my Mom and Dad. Your support is never ending and I have learned so much from you. To all the teachers I have learned from over the years, especially Baron Baptiste, Rolf Gates, Natasha Rizopolous, Ame Wren and Tiffany Cruikshank. And to the people I've shared yoga with over the years in my classes, workshops and trainings: I have learned so much in my working with you and hope we continue to enjoy the journey of yoga together in the years to come.

" ...... We cannot achieve greatness unless we lose all interest in being great. For our own idea of greatness is illusory, and if we pay too much attention to it we will be lured out of the peace and stability of the being God gave us, and seek to live in a myth we have created for ourselves. It is, therefore, a very great thing to be little, which is to say: to be ourselves. And when we are truly ourselves we lose most of the futile self-consciousness that keeps us constantly comparing ourselves with others in order to see how big we are."

Thomas Merton

Preface

When I went to my first teacher training with Baron Baptiste in the summer of 2002, I had no idea I wanted to teach yoga. I had been practicing at the Baptiste studio in Cambridge, MA for about 18 months. My prior experience with yoga before going to the Baptiste studios was only one class I had taken while at a resort in St. Lucia a few months before. I remember being in that first experience and crying most of the time (I had just gone through a divorce). The experience made me inquisitive about yoga in general and a few months later, in December 1999, a few friends, guys actually, told me they'd found a really hard work out. "Heated power yoga," they said and encouraged me to try it. I was going to the gym regularly but was looking for something new.

My first experience was in a class taught by my (now) friend, Coeli Marsh. I remember thinking how impressively she handled the room. It was packed with people of all ages, shapes, sizes and experience levels. She moved with great ease and confidence and presented us with one of the most challenging physical practices I had ever done.

Through that first experience, I was intrigued enough to continue with classes. I found myself going regularly and about a year after my first class, saw a sign for a teacher training. At that point in my corporate career, I was leading a team of people in a health care consulting company. I'd already had exposure to health care, rehabilitation counseling and physical therapy due to my academic and business career thus far. I had no interest in teaching, or so I thought. I figured it'd be a good way to go on vacation and do some yoga.

Well, for anyone that has attended a Baptiste teacher training, led by one of my teachers, Baron Baptiste, it's definitely not a vacation. What it is though, is a physical, spiritual and developmental journey, with the practice and teaching of yoga as a foundation. I could write a whole separate book on my experience in the training and the trainings that followed but suffice it to say upon my return, I started to teach my friend Diane and her girlfriends for free at her home. It was my way to stay committed to developing the skill of yoga teaching. Something had stirred in me at that first training and I wanted to continue to see it through.

I've been teaching ever since I returned from training in August 2002. I taught while working full time, quit my job and taught full time for the Baptiste studios from 2003-2006. I went back to work again and taught part time until I started my own company, Bare Bones Yoga, on September 30, 2010. I had been laid off from my corporate job and decided to take my part time endeavor and make it a full time business.

I wish I would have had a book to guide me through the first few years of teaching, both from a business and teaching perspective. As I gained experience and especially as I developed my own business, I looked for ways to share information in both areas: business and teaching. I started the Bare Bones Yoga Mentorship Program, which allows me to work one-on-one with teachers in individual teaching sessions. I began to write dozens of articles for websites like MindBodyGreen, YOGA-NONYMOUS and DoYogaYoga. I made videos and posted them on my website and YouTube channel. But I wanted to pull all of it together into one place of reference. So, I decided to write this book. It's my way of accumulating all the information in one place and to help those that are thinking of entering this wonderful career of teaching yoga, or already are teaching and have questions about it from the business or teaching perspective. There are so many aspects to it and there can be quite a difference, especially on the business side of things, if you teach full time versus part time. But from the teaching side of things, part time or full time, it's a wonderful way to help people tap into that which is resident within them as a source of strength, relaxation and overall health.

I always tell new teachers that nothing in your life will ever be wasted in the practice of teaching yoga. Whatever you have done in your life before coming to teaching will be useful. You may be a mom or a dad, a corporate businessperson or someone in healthcare. Maybe you're a student or someone that has returned to school after being in the workplace. Maybe you're a massage therapist or a therapist and you're looking for a complementary profession. Everyone that wants to teach yoga comes with academic, work and life experience that can be applied. The piece that is often less understood is the business side of teaching. This was a huge learning curve for me. My 20 plus years of business experience have helped me to apply rules of solid business to my yoga business. Especially for anyone thinking of going into teaching as a full time career, this book will lay out a foundation for you to build this kind of career and lifestyle.

Teaching yoga is not easy. It is a physical job and one that requires your full attention in order to be effective. It requires an ability to be of service to others, regardless of what else is going on in your life. It requires you be responsible, approachable, and steadfast in your commitment to do what needs to be done regardless of distractions and resistance coming at you. It requires you stay true to yourself despite many temptations to do something else, due to outside pressures, lack of self-confidence and lack of experience. It requires courage, for to stand in front of a group of people and lead them through a physical practice means you are willing to show yourself to them. For those that are teaching, you know that the power of connection is found in the ability of the teacher to share from the heart, even if the content of his or her words are on the physical plane. For those reading who are not teaching, you know as we all do, the power of connection found between people when there is authenticity. This is one of the key factors for quality teaching: that innate ability to inspire through command of the information but also through being real and authentic in your presentation.

I hope that you will find this book informative, illuminating and practical. I called it "Stretched" because not only will you stretch your body and mind through the practice, but as a teacher, you will be stretched in ways you never expected - both personally and professionally. Some aspects of this will be uncomfortable at times, but in the end, you will grow in so many ways. I also meant it to be an ongoing reference guide that you can use throughout your career. I wish you all the best on your journey as a yoga teacher.

Namaste.

Karen Fabian
Boston, MA
April 14, 2014

Table of Contents

Business Chapters

Teaching Chapters

Specialty Teaching Chapters

Worksheets, Forms and Documents

Chapter 1

Selecting a Yoga Teacher Training Program that is Right for You

Focus

This chapter provides guidelines for selecting a yoga teacher training program based on the your individual preferences, experiences and plans for teaching. With the popularity of yoga continuing to grow, the proliferation of teacher training programs continues as well. This can make it confusing and overwhelming to try to find a training program that meets your needs.

Overall Considerations

Attending a yoga teacher training program can be a wonderful experience. The opportunity to practice yoga as part of a well-structured intensive can create major shifts in both your body and your mind. Also, for many who attend training as the first step in starting a teacher career, it can provide the critical instruction needed to begin teaching as well as help one start to build a professional network. In order to start the process, let's begin with a few questions that will help determine your background with yoga. These questions are meant to help you start to identify the characteristics of a training program that will meet your needs. Since you're working on these independently, just jot down the answers so you have the history in one place for your review.

Yoga Assessment Questions

- How long have you been practicing yoga?
- What style of yoga do you practice?
- Where do you attend classes?
- What is the reason you'd like to attend a yoga teacher training program?
- What would you like to gain from a yoga teacher training program?
- What is your vision for how you'd like to teach yoga, if at all?

- From a learning perspective, do you prefer small groups or large?
- Do you prefer individual attention or prefer the group dynamic?
- Do you have a full-time job? Describe what you do for work.
- From a lifestyle perspective, share information about your ability to take time off to devote to learning a new craft. Would your lifestyle support a weeklong training, weeknight training over a few weeks or months or would your schedule be more amenable to a highly customized individual program?
- From a timing perspective, what is your desired timeframe to attend training?
- From a location perspective, do you have a preference for local training or one that would require travel outside of your state?
- From a financial perspective, what cost factors do you need to consider in order to make an investment of approximately $3000?

Keep these questions and your answers in mind as you begin to get out there and evaluate programs. Keep these things handy as you talk to people about the programs they attended or talk to teachers about their programs. These are some of the factors to consider consider when selecting a program. Add anything else that you feel is important, such as quality of accommodations for training, time off during training for relaxation and any other items you might consider important.

Strategy

Let's now discuss the overall process to help you select a teacher training program.

Select a Style: The selection of a particular training program should be related to the style of yoga you practice as a student. Often, as you develop a personal practice with a particular teacher and at a particular location, you may begin to develop an interest in attending teacher training. Even if the location you attend for class does not offer training at their location, if they are part of an affiliate program or part of a larger studio system, they may offer a training program. If not, this is the most natural place to start to discuss your intention for training. Ask the studio owner for advice on selecting a training that would be most related to the style of yoga you are practicing at that studio.

Keep in mind that much of your inspiration for teaching will come from your own practice. Attending a training that focuses on a style with which you have no experience can potentially be a waste of your time and money.

Select a Teacher Mentor: Take the time you need to get to know the teacher leading the training. Even within a particular style of yoga, the person leading the training can have his or her own expression of the style. There are so many ways that you can learn about the teacher: all methods of social media, attending local trainings or workshops, books, DVDs, live streaming classes, or regular classes if they are available near you. These are all cost-effective ways you can learn about the teacher and see if his or her style and presentation works for you.

Investigate the format of training: If you prefer personal attention, it might not make sense to attend training where there are lots of people. If you want to learn about the Sutras and traditional yoga philosophy, attending a training that focuses more on yoga sequencing and alignment won't be a good fit. Talk to people that have attended in the past, talk to the yoga teacher's business office and read the descriptions on their website. Look for a posted daily agenda for the training, if there is one, and if there isn't, ask the business office what the daily agenda will include. Closely look at what's included; see if the components are pieces that are interesting to you and part of your overall plan for training.

Recognize that trainings that require travel are not vacations: Along with investigating the format of the training in terms of the presentation of information, it is critical that you understand that teacher training programs are an intense learning experience that often includes self-exploration exercises, sharing and other personal development practice as well as the physical practice. Many times, a student will attend training, ill-prepared for both the physical and mental demands and looking for time to relax. This can often happen at trainings that occur in exotic locations. Please be honest with yourself and if it's a yoga vacation you desire, don't waste your money on a teacher training (unless of course, money is no obstacle).

Establish a regular personal practice: Teacher trainings usually have a strict agenda. They have to; there is a great deal of information to review. As such, they're hard on the body and mind but again, this all comes with the benefit of absorbing valuable teachings and experiences. One of the best preparations you can do before you leave is to develop a habit of practicing. Ideally, you'd have access to a studio that supports the style of yoga that will be the focus of the teacher training, but even if not, just be practicing daily or at least 3 days a week. This will create a strong body, which you'll need for the extensive practices you'll do at training. This will also create the discipline you'll need to leverage when you're hard at work at training.

Prepare to give of yourself 100%: Teacher trainings are the magical combination of wisdom meeting intellect, soul meeting intelligence, the group experience supporting the individual, which in turn, supports the group. These trainings can be transformative if everyone is there giving of themselves fully. This means in each interaction with others, in providing feedback, in participating in different exercises, do it completely. It means being present, without distractions. The more you are there for the others, the more they can be there for you. That all contributes to an amazing experience for everyone.

Cost Considerations: Teacher training programs can cost anywhere from $1500 to a few thousand dollars. Generally, training programs run approximately $2500 and, for those that require travel, do not include flight costs but may involve lodging and food. Most, if not all programs require a deposit by a certain date to hold your spot. This also gives the teacher a chance to determine interest. They then provide you with a payment schedule, including when the final payment is required.

Many programs will not return your deposit, even if you cancel for any reason. Be very careful to read ALL the disclaimers on their website and any contract you are asked to sign, be sure to understand what you may lose financially if you have to cancel. Some training programs may allow a refund if there is an emergency, but this may be totally at their discretion.

Time Considerations: Training programs are usually formatted as either "destination trainings," where you travel to a location to attend training or a local training, where you attend a local studio site for training. Trainings in off-site locations are usually one week long but can be as long as one month and can occur in destinations like Bali or

India.

Local trainings are often conducted during several weekends and may include some weeknights. These trainings are often for those who cannot fit a destination training into their schedule but may involve late week nights and entire weekends devoted to training.

As with all factors, be honest with yourself about what is best for you logistically and also what will provide you with a format that will allow you to be present and prepared to learn. If you have a stressful job and home situation, perhaps finding a way to take a week off will give you a better chance to devote yourself to learning instead of trying to apply yourself to learning yoga after a full week of work.

Medical, Mental or other Physical Considerations to consider: Please be sure that before you attend any intensive on yoga teaching, that you are in good physical health. The energy necessary to learn and be part of the team of teacher trainees will come from your physical and mental resources.

Also, while yoga is a wonderful practice, both on the physical and mental level, many yoga teacher trainings will require you do an in-depth personal exploration to understand more about yourself. While this may be a wonderful way to work through some existing mental blocks, it may not be the place to work through existing and current challenges. If you have any concerns, you should discuss them with both your medical professionals as well as the teacher training team before you attend training.

Also, a few side notes: if you are taking any medication for any issue, many trainings will ask that you disclose this as part of their application process. Also, the physical demands of training can be significant, especially if you attend a week-long intensive. Further, if the training is in an exotic location, access to medical care may be limited. This is not to scare you, but to be sure you are prepared for what's ahead and can enjoy your training.

Think ahead: Plan some time when you get home to transition back to a normal schedule. You'll not only need your rest; you'll need time to re-adjust to, in many cases, a regular sleep schedule, a regular eating routine and, more importantly, you'll need time to give your heart and soul time to absorb everything that you've learned. Much of it will be intellectual but much of it will be about you, your abilities, what you want to do with your future and identifying what you're passionate about.

Online Resources: Both Yoga Alliance (www.yogaalliance.org) and Yoga Journal (www.yogajournal.com) have excellent website directories to help you find a school. While searching online for a training program is one approach, it is always helpful to have personal contact with the school and the teachers through participation in classes, workshops and events.

Closing Summary

Teacher training is a wonderful way to start on your path to teaching. Once you have completed this chapter, you will be on your way to making a selection of a program.

Chapter 2

Understanding the Yoga Industry

Focus

This chapter will provide an understanding of the components of the yoga industry, including an understanding of Yoga Alliance, the concept of "certification", employment status, and other employment information (including information about taxes and health insurance). This will help a teacher navigate the industry and make knowledgeable decisions about investing in trainings, programs and business infrastructure.

Overall Considerations

As a yoga teacher, especially a new teacher entering the business, there are several considerations to take into account at the start. These things fall into certain categories, all having an effect on both the set up and the cost of maintaining your business. Even for teachers that teach full-time for a studio and have all their classes in that one location, there are still things to be considering around the insurance, taxes and certification.

Many of these features are still in development as the industry matures. The role of Yoga Alliance, for instance, has grown over the past several years and it is now a recognized piece of the yoga industry. Other components, like the idea of aligning with a certain teacher and style of yoga, has been around longer.

All the decisions a teacher makes around these components involve time and money, which as a teacher, are valuable commodities. Therefore, the more you know as a teacher, the more informed you'll be around how you use your precious resources.

The formal yoga industry consists of studios and teachers all over the world. Each studio runs independently, although there are studio systems that are comprised of studios in different locations that are all part of the same Registered Yoga School (RYS). There are many independent studios that stand alone and are not part of any larger system as well and there are studios that are "affiliates," which is a status granted by some RYS to other studios that teach the same style, are staffed with teachers that have gone through the same program and have met certain other standards set by the main RYS.

As a Yoga Teacher, you are an independent contractor and you may carry individual certifications and/or registration through Yoga Alliance (see next section). Teachers are mostly free agents, with freedom to pursue teaching opportunities anywhere they'd like. As a result, they have the ability to work in studios, gyms and other existing locations that offer yoga. However, they also have the freedom to create programs of their own and bring yoga to locations that may currently not have a yoga program.

*Special note: When you take a teaching job, find out if the studio owner has any concerns about you teaching in other locations close to their site. It is always better to have this conversation up front. The more experienced and the greater your role as a teacher on the studio schedule, the studio may ask you sign a non-compete contract, which is meant to protect them in the event you leave and take a new job in another studio that is close to their site. This might result in their students following you to your new location so the non-compete is there in an effort for them to protect their business. It can also require that as long as you are teaching for that one location, you can't take any jobs within a certain mile radius from the studio.

The yoga industry has a few recognized industry magazines, such as Yoga Journal and Yoga International. There are also several conferences held by Yoga Journal for purposes of networking and offering continuing education to teachers in the form of classes and lectures.

The yoga industry works largely on the concept of networking, with teachers finding jobs and other opportunities by creating networks of friends and business colleagues. It will be critical for you as a new teacher to create a business network that you can lean on for growth of your business.

Training, Certification and Yoga Alliance Registration

Before you started your yoga-training program, you most likely did some research on which training program to select. Your choice might have been influenced by the teacher, the location or even the format for the training in terms of the schedule or what was included in the training program.

Once you complete your training, you should receive a document that indicates the program you completed, when you started and finished and the name of the program. Some programs might also give you a designation you can use after your name to indicate you completed the training. This might be something like "Certified (XXXX) Teacher," where XXXX refers to the name of the program you completed. Other programs may not indicate a title you have been awarded but may give you the certificate to use as proof of completion.

Why does this matter? This kind of factor matters only as much as you feel it is an important factor in relation to your work as a yoga teacher. The kind of program you completed will give students a way to recognize you and the style of yoga you teach. The title you are given upon completion (if there is one) will be used in your marketing materials, website and in any place that your name appears (or it should). This may provide you with some validity and recognition when it comes to others having an understanding of the kind of training you received.

*Special note: Some programs are very specific with regard to how you can use their name in your title. Be sure you understand any restrictions around the use of the name of the program you completed after your name.

Yoga training programs are usually a significant investment in terms of cost and time. Some programs, while shorter and handled on a remote basis, may differ in cost and length of time but most in-person training programs require a significant investment. As such, it is not unreasonable to expect that you would receive something in exchange for your time and effort. Some programs will also include you on their website as part of a "Teacher Listing." This is also something that is helpful to know before you complete a program. Being listed in this way can lead to new business opportunities for you, as people browsing the website find you.

Certification

As discussed above, upon completion, some programs will provide you with the title, "Certified XXXX Teacher" when you are done. If so, you should use this in all places where your name appears. Be sure that when someone else does any marketing for you or creates materials (either in print or on the internet) that your name and title appear correctly (including spelling of your program name).

The concept of "Certification" is recognition by the Teacher of the training program that you have completed the program and he or she endorses you as a teacher able to provide yoga services according to his or her standards. Certification is only offered by individual teachers or schools and is not something you are able to obtain by belonging to Yoga Alliance. Certification indicates a close affiliation of some sort with the certifying body, either by completing a certain number of hours of training and/ or by also completing other training components such as hours of teaching, readings, essay and other writing, teaching classes under the guidance and supervision of a more senior teacher in the program or any other requirement that the specific school or founder of the program requires.

Certification is not a guarantee of quality and does not provide a student with guaranteed assurance that their classroom experience will meet their needs or be safe or what they expected. However, the more extensive the program requirements, the smaller the training programs, the more experience and requirements held out for aspiring teachers, the more confident a yoga consumer of services can be that the teacher is well trained and qualified to teach yoga. Shorter programs and especially those that are offered remotely provide more of a challenge around ensuring quality simply because yoga as a modality is best taught in person. However, this by no means is an overall position and there are many people with related certifications that learn yoga in this way.

Yoga Alliance

Yoga Alliance is a non-profit business that was formed in 1999 and according to their mission statement are a "national education and support organization who works in the public interest to ensure there is a thorough understanding of the benefits of yoga, that the teachers of yoga value its history and traditions and that the public can be confident of the quality and consistency of instruction." Yoga Alliance offers a "Registration" which is different from being a "Certified" teacher. Being "Registered" means that you have completed a 200 Hour or 500 Hour program with a yoga school that has been designated by Yoga Alliance as a recognized school. Yoga Alliance has developed standards that they believe ensure quality and integrity around the provision of yoga services and yoga studios apply to YA to receive the designation "Registered Yoga School" (RYS).

If you attend a training program given by one of these RYS, you receive the designation of "Registered Yoga Teacher" at either the 200 or 500-hour level, depending on the program you completed. With additional teaching experience, you can also attain the designation "Experienced Registered Yoga Teacher," which acknowledges that you've taught at least 1000 hours in addition to completing the RYS's program.

In order to get your Registration status with YA, you must fill out registration information on the Yoga Alliance website, pay the annual fee and in exchange, they will list you on their website. This is another way that potential students can locate you.

In order to maintain your Registration status, every 3 years you must submit to YA the hours of continuing education work you have completed. They require 45 teaching hours and 30 training hours. For all details on registering and requirements and to find RYS, see www. yogaalliance.org.

Employment Information

There are a number of things to consider from an employment perspective when considering becoming a yoga teacher. Yoga teachers are generally independent contractors although in some circumstances, they are actually employees paid after filling out a W-4 form. This is rare, as most studios don't take on the job of withholding taxes from your pay. If you are an independent contractor, you must take on the responsibility of setting aside money for federal and state income taxes.

If you teach in a gym or have created your own opportunity for teaching, let's say in a non-profit, it is possible that you will fill out a W-4 form and the employer will take taxes out of your paycheck. However, as stated above, this is rare.

As an independent contractor, you will set aside money out of your pay and use it for the tax payment on April 15 or you will pre-pay your taxes over the course of 4 payments done quarterly. Throughout the year, track your earned income via a spreadsheet that captures all of your earnings. At the end of the year, you will use this total annual income figure to calculate your tax payment to the Federal and Local government. If you don't set money aside or pre-pay, it is likely, depending on how much you make that you will have a significant bill from the Federal and State government to pay.

It is very important for any job opportunity that you secure, that you ask before you start what the pay situation is like. Find out how you will be paid, if taxes are withheld and what forms you need to fill out. Be clear with your hiring contact as to the tax arrangement so you can know what your obligations are regarding taxes.

As an independent contractor, you will also carry your own liability insurance. This protects you at any location where you teach. Although the claim would need to be accepted by the carrier for coverage to apply (as with any form of insurance), the coverage is to protect you from any lawsuit brought on by a student who claims injury as a result of your teaching.

As an independent contractor, you should also carry your own health insurance. While it can be expensive, when you work for a living using your body as part of your teaching, it's critical that you have coverage for treatment in case of injury. If you can't work, you don't get paid. Even if you have purchased disability insurance, it will only cover you for a portion of your earnings. Understand that generally speaking, employers do not provide health insurance coverage to teachers. In some rare instances, if you work for a location that has you on staff as a team member, like a gym for instance, you may be offered health insurance but again, this is very rare. As purchasing health insurance as an individual can be very expensive, it is important that you recognize this as part of the expense of being a yoga teacher. The task of finding your own health insurance is a separate topic and varies from state to state in terms of available options, although now with federally mandated health care, anyone can get an insurance plan through the Affordable Care Act. If you wish to purchase in the private market but don't want or can't afford individual rates, you can look for group rates. As a small business owner, you may be able to join a local chapter of the Small Business Association and use that membership to buy insurance under a group rate. Also, Yoga Alliance has begun to offer group rates for insurance.

As an independent contractor, it is very important to keep good records. You'll want a record of your revenue earned, what revenue was taxed and what revenue was not, and you'll want to track all your expenses as much of it can be deducted when you do your taxes. (the chapter, "Building the Infrastructure of your Yoga-preneurship" will help you with tools and processes to track this information).

Closing Summary

The yoga industry is ever changing and moving in many directions. You will have many opportunities to grow as a teacher and the more you can define the directions you'd like to pursue and follow up diligently, the more you'll create a fulfilling career for yourself.

Chapter 3

Getting Started Once You've Completed Your 200-hour Program

Focus

Once you graduate from your Teacher Training program, chances are, you'll want to get started right away. With some luck and good planning, you'll most likely have your first teaching gig already in place and ready to start once you're done. If not, review the chapter on "Identifying and Evaluating Yoga Teaching Opportunities and Pricing your Classes" to find your first job.

Also, by the time you're ready to teach your first class, the assumption is you've already set your rate for teaching, negotiated that rate with the studio owner, have confirmed what you'll be paid and how and have set up the necessary spreadsheets to track classes taught and your expenses. If not, review the chapter on "Building the Infrastructure of your Yoga-Preneurship" and be sure that you have this all in place. Also, be sure to have your teaching insurance in place.

While training programs are great for giving you the knowledge and information you'll need to teach a class, they may not cover what to do before you teach your first class. There are critical steps you'll need to take in order to ensure that your transition to teaching is smooth, effective and professional.

Overall Considerations

Get your certificate from the Teacher Training Program you've completed and start your Continuing Education Folder.

Your Teacher Training Program will give you a certificate to indicate that you graduated and will include the dates of attendance and the name of the school itself. Once you receive this, make a few color copies and get them either laminated or protect them in a folder or clear cover. Secondly, start a folder where you'll keep all documents related to completed trainings. Over the years, as you complete more training, it's helpful to have all these documents in one place.

Submit your information to Yoga Alliance to become registered as a Yoga Teacher

Most of the yoga schools conducting training are registered as yoga schools with Yoga Alliance. This is not always the case but you probably checked this out before you attended the training. If your school is registered, you can go online to the Yoga Alliance website (www.yogaalliance.org) and submit your graduation information so you can become a Registered Yoga Teacher.

Registering with Yoga Alliance will establish your teaching credentials as an "R.Y.T." which stands for a Registered Yoga Teacher. Many yoga schools are registered and as a result of attending their recognized training, you are a Registered Yoga Teacher. You can use this designation on your teaching resume and website. Some studios will require you have the R.Y.T. designation in order to be employed. Others will not.

Get your liability insurance

It's critical you have liability insurance. This protects you when teaching and most studios will ask that you provide a copy of this document. One company that provides insurance is Philadelphia Insurance Company (www.phly.com) but there are others as well.

The cost of this insurance is minimal when compared to the dollar limits provided in coverage. Once you receive this coverage statement (especially if it's emailed to you versus mailed), be sure to print or copy the coverage page (it will be a large document but the first few pages are the important ones) and include this in your folder (as above). You will pay them annually (keep a copy of your check and statement for tax purposes).

Create your Yoga Resume

Even for new teachers that have not yet begun to teach, there is much that can be included on a resume. Include your professional experience, but slant the content towards skills that can be transferred to teaching. Include your training and its focus and a statement about your teaching style.

This document should be kept in a folder in hard copy. It should also be kept in a folder on your computer with your biography (see below for how to build that). You'll keep updating it as you gain more experience. This also will contain the items you'll add to your Linked In profile. (you'll have to decide if you want one Linked In profile for your professional career and one for your teaching career).

If you're looking for specific help with building a resume, see the chapter on "Resume Creation and Marketing."

Write your biography paragraph and submit to the studio owner for posting on their website

Most studios will post your picture and biography on their website. These items should be standard files you have on your computer and can access immediately. I cannot tell you how impressed studio owners will be if you can respond immediately to a request for both. Studio owners are usually covering many things and when they have a moment to post your information, you don't want them to be waiting for your data.

Your biography should include the style of yoga you teach, the name of the teacher who led your training, your website (if you have one) and a few personal things about yourself so people can get an idea of who you are as a person. Any personal stories about how you started with yoga are great from the perspective of building a connection with students. If you had a back injury, for instance, and that was the catalyst to start yoga and now you're a teacher, this can be a huge factor to encourage people to attend your classes if they are experiencing a similar thing.

Write your class description and post on the studio website

Just as the studio will ask you for a biography, they will most likely ask you to contribute to or write the description for your class. If they don't, you absolutely want to be sure the description being used is accurate and reflects what you'll be presenting.

The class description should include the style of yoga that will be presented but remember that many people are not familiar with Sanskrit. Use English and words that are understandable by anyone. Things like "Vinyasa" and "Yin" may be accurate but many won't understand what they mean. Include them, but add a few statements that outline what people can expect.

Include a statement about the experience level needed for class. If your class is focused on the basics or more appropriate for beginners, have the name reflect that. If it's a class open to any level of student, say that. If you're a teacher who routinely offers handstands or headstands, write that too. Be honest so people know what to expect.

One special note: if the class will be heated, be sure the description reflects that and add some other suggestions about what to wear and to bring a towel and water.

Take a few professional headshots and yoga pose photographs and submit one to the studio's owner for posting on their website

It's worth the investment to have a professional take your picture. You should have some in which you can clearly see your face and you're not in a pose and some where you are in a few yoga poses. Think about the image you wish to project and your style of teaching. If you want to present as a person who teaches classes that are highly accessible, doing a split may not be the pose you wish to do. Also, if you have your own brand name, wear a piece of clothing that has the name to create brand awareness.

These pictures will be used in a variety of ways. You'll need them to post on your website, studio websites, for use in promotional posters and for use on social media. Also, one note about professional protocol: if you use pictures of you teaching in class, be sure to get the agreement of the people in class to use the pictures in any social media or promotional posts. Or, at a minimum, before you take the shot, let people know you're taking some pictures so anyone that does not want to be in the shot has a chance to step away. Also, be very judicious about using pictures of children in promotional postings. If you can get the agreement of the parents or caregivers, this goes a long way to acknowledging you plan to use the pictures for promotion. Also, you can take pictures of children from the back so you can't see their faces.

Check all the data about you and your classes on the studio's website before teaching your first class

Before you teach your first class, check the studio website and be sure that your name, the title of the class, the description and the time and length of class are all correct. This is a good idea as sometimes there can be errors in the translation from your documents and what was posted.

Get your CPR and first aid Certification from your local Red Cross

Just as if you were a teacher in a school or in any other job where you're leading a group experience, you should have CPR and First Aid training. This gives you the essential steps you'll need to take should one of your students have a medical issue in class. Keep in mind that many times, you'll be the only person in the studio at the time of your class (many studios do not provide assistants or front desk coverage while you're teaching). In this case, you need to be confident that if an issue arises, you'll be calm and able to direct others in the class to assist so you can stay with the injured party.

Make a copy of your CPR card and keep it in the folder with your professional documents, like your resume and teaching certificate. Studios may ask for verification that you have completed this training.

Have professional yoga clothing you'll wear to teach

What you wear to teach may be different from what you wear to practice. While you may love a certain pair of pants and low cut or midriff tops or love that comfy yoga shirt that has the holes in it, this isn't what you should wear to teach.

When you teach, you need to ensure you can move around the room and assist students without having any concern about your clothes falling off, slipping off the shoulders or tripping you. You also want to ensure you blend and are not a distraction to the class. This doesn't mean you can't wear what you like but you should use discretion and remember that being professional is an important piece.

Your clothes may also be a distinguishing factor for you. If you like a particular style of clothes, brand or type of jewelry, this can be something you wear consistently that can help you stand out as a teacher. Before you start teaching in your first classes, think about what you might like to portray as a style and stick with it. Think of Hulk Hogan's bandana, Kenny Chesney's cowboy hat and Richard Simmons' tank tops and shorts; these are the stuff of their brand and people always associate one with the other. This is your chance to be creative, individual, and unique and to express yourself!

If you find that you don't have anything in your closet that meets any of these criteria, go shopping! Keep the receipts and use them to submit with your taxes. These clothes are now professional expense deductions (note: some yoga retailers will provide discounts to teachers).

Create a spreadsheet of professional contacts

Start a spreadsheet of contacts in the yoga industry. Include your colleagues from training, teachers you've met, people you admire. If your list is short, start networking! Look for new studios to visit, local workshops to attend and ask people to lunch.

Start assisting on a regular basis

I think this is one of the most important things that new teachers can do in order to keep active, keep learning, gain experience, network with other teachers, learn alignment, observe experienced teachers and be "of service" (among lots of other benefits). Ask your local studio (or the host of your teacher training) if you can assist in classes. If yes, be ready to commit to a regular class on a regular basis.

Assisting should be viewed as a responsibility, not a "do it once every once in a while" kind of thing. If you don't think you have the time to commit long term, at least commit to a few months. The requirement to "show up," regardless of your personal life, your schedule, your attitude that day and how you're feeling is all part of teaching and assisting. You won't be paid but you might gain credits for free classes and you gain tons of experience you can add to your resume.

Practice teaching

One of the hardest things to do once you're done but one of the THE most important things is to start teaching right away. The mental challenge of assimilating all you have learned on an intellectual level and start to express that while also allowing some of yourself to shine through is a big step but will only get harder the longer you wait.

If you don't have a teaching job lined up when you graduate, create opportunities to teach. Get a group of your friends together and teach for free. Ask your local civic or neighborhood groups if they'd like to set up a few free yoga classes. Ask your local Mother's Association if you can do a few sessions for the mothers.

Set up a regular practice schedule at your home based studio

With all the focus on learning, don't forget that being a student of yoga is a huge part of your training. It's also a great way to network and meet other yoga teachers. If you don't have a studio that was the host of your training (and is your 'home base' for your practice), find one. And, if you have a studio at which you'd like to teach, start practicing there. You'll make connections with everyone from the person that does check in to the teachers and clients. Becoming a "known entity" is a big part of getting hired for a teaching job. While you're building connections, you're also practicing yoga.

If there are teachers from whom you wish to learn, visit their classes. There are many master level experienced teachers who offer classes at studios in their home-based towns when they are not traveling. Now that you're done with your training, take the time to explore other teachers and styles. There is much to learn in yoga and nothing you do will be wasted time.

Have a go-to sequence that you'll use for your classes

As a new teacher, you'll have a lot to manage, in addition to your own feelings of fear and nervousness. The last think you'll want to be thinking about is the sequence. Have one you can use regularly and stick to it. You'll become more proficient at it as will your students.

Make it highly accessible and offer modifications throughout. Get used to using essential language so it's understandable by anyone, regardless of yoga experience. Practice it yourself, ask your friends to meet you at your home and do it with them for free. See the chapter on "Using Essential Yoga Language" to get practical tips about teaching in class.

Record yourself teaching (better yet, make a teaching video)

We all have a certain perception of the way we look when teaching. But there's nothing like taping your voice or taking a video of yourself teaching in class. I have a teaching module where I do this with teachers and then we review it for feedback and modification. There is much we communicate with our bodies and much that we say without words. We really can't see this until we literally "see" how we look. We can communicate openness, a willingness to help, confidence, shyness, fear and disapproval all without saying a word. Of course, we want to exude positive vibes but many times our life history, habits and fears get in the way. Taping yourself and working with an experienced teacher for feedback will give you the information you need so you can see clearly and will also give you the tools so you can make positive changes.

To do this, let the class know that someone will be taping the class. Have this person in the back and focusing on you and less on the students. Let the students know that the tape will only be used by you and not for promotional purposes and if anyone wishes to avoid being recorded, move them to a place in the room where they will not be taped.

Steps to take before teaching your first class

Clear your schedule so you have a free hour before your class

When you start teaching that first weekly class, you'll be nervous and you'll want time to relax. You'll also want ample time to get to the studio and park if needed (depending on how you get to class and the distance from your starting point, you may need more than an hour). Set yourself up to be connected to your body by giving yourself enough time. Make sure you do this each week; not just before your very first class.

Another thing to think about is to take care of yourself. Make sure you're hydrated, you've eaten but aren't too full and you're healthy. Don't teach if you're sick or not feeling well. Make sure your hands are clean and so are you.

Find out if you will have someone to check in the students for your class

Not every studio provides a person to do check in when you teach. Be sure it's clear before you teach if you will have someone to do check in for your class. If not, it's important you know how to do check in at the desk.

If you haven't received training, the studio should provide you with it. This process can be a bit unnerving and can create stress you before you teach. Keep in mind that the goal is to get people into the room with as little complication as possible. If you have students with questions about payment or any other administrative issue, make a note of it and let them know you'll have the studio manager contact them. This will create a smooth flow of people into the room and prevent a back up at the desk. This also minimizes controversy; students sometimes have questions about their account, how many classes are left on their card, credits for class, expiring Group On and other deals and all these conversations take time away from the main goal: to get people on their mats with as little stress as possible. Your role as the teacher is not to resolve these issues but to pass the information through to the manager so he or she can resolve it (unless it's your studio, but even in that case, save those conversations for a separate time).

Once you're done with check-in, take a few minutes to clear the desk of anything left from the process. This will give you a few moments to relax and take a few deep breaths. It also will tidy things up for the next person that has to check people in.

If you need to check people into class, be at the studio at least one half hour before. This could be longer depending on how packed the classes get and how early people typically show up. If you are not doing check in, it's a good idea to be inside the studio at least 15 minutes before class so you have a few minutes to check out the room and check for new students on the class roster.

Things to consider before you start teaching your first classes

Music: Music can be a wonderful addition to your classes but it is another variable to manage. The less you give yourself to do, the more energy and attention you can give your students.

Readings: Readings are another addition to your classes that can be really wonderful. It can inspire, inform as well as educate. However, again, this is another variable. It's time you'll be taking before class to select a reading when it might be more helpful to practice yoga yourself so you can be connected to your body.

Themes: Classes built on themes can help students learn new poses and alignment. Some themes for class build on a particular physical concept, such as "Poses to Open the Hips" or "Arm Balances." Other themes may be more spiritual and the teacher may present a string of related thoughts all around a particular idea, such as non-violence or practicing with compassion. While these kinds of classes can be wonderful for both students and teachers, as a beginning teacher, it can be helpful to stick with the same sequence to become more proficient at it (as stated above).

Complex Poses such as Arm Balances and Inversions: While these can be fun to teach, they're not always accessible for many students. Also, to support students as they try more challenging postures, it can be helpful if you have an assistant in class.

Hours of preparation including writing new sequences in a notebook, notes to yourself as to music, themes or any of the other items above: Many new teachers labor for hours before each class, planning, writing and analyzing how they will teach that day. While this shows great dedication and commitment to your craft, it's exhausting and can take you out of your center versus being more prepared to teach.

If you follow the tips above, especially the suggestion that you use the same sequence each time, refrain from using music or themes, you will feel more prepared when you arrive to teach. Changing these variables every time is not only confusing to you but also to your students.

Please keep in mind that just because I'm suggesting you hold off on changing the sequence does not mean that you might not make little variations from time to time in a few sections of the sequence. This may mean in the balancing series you add a pose. It could mean in the hip series at the end of class, you add in a different seated posture. There are many ways to create slight variations without having to spend hours preparing before each class.

Things to be ready to do when class is done

Stay after class

Just as you want time before class to prepare and come into your body, you'll want time after your class to be available to answer questions. Answering student questions is a great way to get to know them, support them and become a resource. Remember that if you are asked something you don't know, say so and follow up in the next class with the answer.

Be a help to set up and break down

Taking a few minutes before and after your class to help set up the room and put away props afterwards will help you be seen as a team member who is willing to help out on many levels. It also communicates to the students that you care about the studio and want it to look clean and neat for everyone. Yoga practice is not just expressed through the poses; it is also expressed through how we care for the space in which we practice.

Closing Summary

The beginning of your teaching career will be filled with excitement and fear. Being organized and controlling what you can, i.e. being on time, being prepared, being well rested and knowing your sequence will all help you focus on being of service to the people around you.

Chapter 4

Building the Infrastructure of Your Yoga-Preneurship

Focus

To provide practical information to help a new yoga teacher set up the infrastructure of his or her yoga business. Tools are included that will help you track expenses, revenue, classes, daily activities, business leads and write a weekly progress report.

Overall Considerations

Completing yoga teacher training is a wonderful accomplishment. Teacher training programs vary in their focus, size, style of presentation and information presented. However, regardless of their particular emphasis, what often is lacking is the practical information to help teachers get started as a teacher. Training programs focus primarily on the teaching aspect of yoga; they may not focus on the business aspects of teaching beyond perhaps a few hours discussing it. Furthermore, each teacher's situation will be very different. In order to get the customized support needed, many teachers either seek out the help they need from a mentor, create the tracking tools on their own, network with other teachers or don't do anything until they realize they need information and don't have what they need.

Having solid skills around tracking certain key pieces of data along with setting business goals, tracking leads, documenting progress towards goals, making revenue projections, tracking expenses, setting goals around additional training and creating a focus for your teaching is all part of developing a discipline around the business aspect of teaching yoga. The assumption we are making, for the purposes of this section, is that you are teaching full time and that teaching is your primary source of income (if you are working part-time in an unrelated role to raise additional money, that is fine). But this program assumes that working as a yoga teacher is a full time endeavor. However, even if you are teaching part-time, many of these tools and discussion points will be applicable.

Paying attention to the detail of your yoga teaching career asks that you treat it as a business; that it's not a passing endeavor that you are doing "until something else comes along." While it takes more time to go through these steps, once you have much of the infrastructure built, it actually frees you up to teach, because you're not worrying about if your bills will be paid on time or if you remember to get a sub for that class you have to skip next week or will you have the data ready for your accountant so that you can file your taxes on time. It's wonderful to connect to all the good and spiritual aspects of yoga, but it's very hard to enjoy any of that in your classes if your personal business life is falling apart.

So, make the commitment to spend the time to set up your business, and you'll have more time to spend teaching. Furthermore, it's not as challenging to keep track of things when your schedule is light and you're just starting out; but you want your business to grow from a teaching and revenue perspective. Having these tools in place will allow you to seamlessly increase your productivity and still keep track of key data points.

Let's begin with a review of the key points in setting up your business:

Begin with the end in mind. This wonderful concept from Stephen Covey's book, "The Seven Habits of Highly Effective People," suggests that for any project, any business and really, for your life, you begin with an idea of how you want things to end. As it relates to our lives, we might think, "I want to die a happy person." Well, each day, you then know that happiness is your primary goal. Now, that is an overly simplistic and not very specific goal, but you get the idea.

As it relates to being a yoga teacher, these days there are many ways to apply your skills as a teacher. Just some of the variables include the training you selected, the style of yoga you are going to teach, the setting, the typical clientele, the age of your typical student. The assumption is you selected and completed a teacher training that takes into account some of the above considerations. But beyond the training, here are some other things to consider:

42

- How do you wish to apply this training?
- Where do you see yourself teaching?
- Why kinds of students do you wish to teach?
- Do you primarily want to teach in studios?
- Do you want to teach in a number of studios or just one or a few?
- Do you want to teach for one business/studio system or many?
- Do you want to offer workshops?
- Do you want to offer teacher trainings?
- Do you wish to offer retreats?
- Do you want to develop your own yoga brand?
- Do you want to teach specialty groups, like children, mothers and babies, teens?
- Do you want to offer other non-teaching wellness support, like wellness coaching?
- Do you want to offer other non-teaching business services like writing wellness articles, doing speaking engagements?

Identify what your ultimate yoga business model looks like. Don't worry if you're not sure of all the pieces. Just begin with some statements that describe how you wish your business to look. Beginning with this overall statement will give you something to check back against as you begin doing things at the day-to-day level.

Note: There may be times you specifically decide to branch out in an unrelated area that is not related to your overall vision. This may be because you want to try a new teaching skill or want to investigate a new angle or simply need the money. This is fine. But keep in mind what your overall vision is for your business and let that shape the leads you pursue, the jobs you take and the brand, if any, that you develop for your business.

Set up your Business Dashboard (see included spreadsheet in final section). This will become your master spreadsheet that you use to track your business leads. It will contain:

- A tab that outlines your overall vision from an "activity" and "projected revenue" perspective (Activity/Revenue)
- A tab that tracks your overall revenue from week to week (Actual Revenue)
- Individual tabs that reflect the different business verticals that you

are pursuing. For instance, one tab might be for studio teaching, one for privates, one for children's yoga and one for speaking engagements.

Decide what you need to earn (revenue target) in order to break even (earnings= expenses). Then, increase that number by some factor. This is your Dream Big Number! It might be 10% more, it might be 50% more. Think big! Only by thinking big will you begin to act big. It's not so much that you know exactly how you're going to get there; it's more that you begin to get your brain into the habit of believing that your business will work and more than just get by, it will do exceptionally well! This is positive thinking at work, but it's part of an entire business model. So, rather than depending on positive thoughts alone, it's positive thoughts coupled with good planning. That is an unbeatable combination for success (more on this in the book "The Secret", in the chapter on money).

Know your Dream Big Daily Number. This is your daily revenue target. This is derived by taking your Dream Big Number, dividing it by 12 (months), then by 4 (weeks) and then taking that number and dividing by 5, 6 or 7 (days). This number is your daily revenue target. It doesn't make much sense to divide by 7 because you want to give yourself at least one day off. Keep in mind that some days you'll make much more, if you have special events or trainings. Some days, you'll make nothing or less than the number. But having this number in mind helps you understand how things are going each day as you're teaching; it helps you better evaluate each opportunity as it comes up; helps you set your rate per transaction and gives you a target to shoot for on a daily basis.

Identify the teaching and non-teaching wellness opportunities you need to book in order to reach your Dream Big Number. This number will go at the top of your Activity/Revenue tab of your Business Dashboard. Then, you'll list on this tab the actual activities and how many of them you'll need to hit this number.

Note: You may find, as you are going through this exercise that you need to book many classes a week in order to hit even your break even number. If that is the case, you need to identify other teaching gigs that have the potential to pay more per transaction. This specific topic is discussed in greater detail in another chapter, "Identifying and Evaluating Yoga Teaching Opportunities/Pricing Classes", but suffice it to say teaching privates and non-studio gigs have greater potential for you to make money than teaching studio classes (with the exception of teacher trainings and workshops you hold at a studio).

Create a spreadsheet to track revenue. This will allow you to easily keep track of every teaching activity you do, where, how much you were paid, if it was taxed, if not, what percentage you are setting aside for taxes, the hours you taught and any comments about the class. This becomes critical when you need to submit hours to Yoga Alliance or get a quick snapshot of revenue earned per year. Get into the habit of opening up this sheet every day and logging your classes. Do not wait until the end of the week! This should be part of your daily routine.

Create a spreadsheet to track expenses. Track what you bought, where and the method of payment. Be sure to include a column for "Category" so at the end of the year, it's easy for your accountant to do your taxes. Include things like transportation, airfare, clothing, books.

Use your Business Dashboard to track leads and their individual status. In the first section, we talked about setting up separate tabs that represent your individual business verticals (categories). Start building these business verticals by going into each tab and identifying leads for each vertical. For instance, if one tab is for "Studios," write down all the studios where you wish to pursue teaching and indicate in a Status column the status of your contact with that studio. Make a column for "Contact Person" and "Phone Number." Then, any time you have a call or exchange emails with this lead in an effort to secure a job there, you can update this entry. This allows you to have one place of reference for all your leads and decreases the chance that you'll have to sort through old emails to follow up.

Open a business bank account with a checking and savings account. This should be done right away. Part of having your own business is setting up a separate account into which you'll deposit your earnings. Even if you're paid cash for something, rather than put the money in your wallet, deposit it. It builds the discipline of keeping your "earnings" separate from your "living money" and it allows you to track revenue from your business easily. It's also helpful to have your business account in the same bank as your personal account. That way, you can transfer money electronically to "Pay Yourself" for personal expenses and savings.

Pay yourself first! This concept, from the book, "The Automatic Millionaire", is an important one and even more important when you are working for yourself. As a self-employed person, you need to set up many of the functions that corporate workers have handled for them by their employers. Taking care of health insurance, saving for your retirement and putting aside money for taxes is all your responsibility. It's so easy to be caught up in all that has to be paid out that you can forget that the first person that should be paid is YOU! If you create this infrastructure and simply give all your money away you will be frustrated quickly and will feel like you're simply treading water. "But I don't make enough to save any money yet," you might say. This is simply not true. The ACT of saving is more important than how much you save. In saving money, what we're doing is building the discipline to save weekly; you're rewarding and acknowledging oneself for a job well done and from a practical standpoint, we're building a nest egg for emergencies and additional expenses. This transaction can easily be done electronically by making a weekly transfer from your business account to your personal savings account of some percentage of your weekly earnings. Again, maybe it's only a small amount, but because it's a percentage of your weekly earnings, it will increase as you earn more. Don't make the transfer automatic; actually log into your online bank account and move the money yourself. You'll feel so good when you do (and there will be a note on your Daily Worksheet to remind you to make this transfer weekly – more on that later).

Use your business savings account to save money to pay your taxes. One of the critical things for yoga teachers is to save money for taxes. Many other kinds of business owners have to make estimated tax payments. This is a hard but necessary discipline to which you must commit. Estimate what your tax liability will be (even use last year's return as a benchmark, unless you expect to earn a lot more in the first year of your business or something else significant has changed in your financial picture). Determine how this tax liability breaks down when you divide it up over the year or as a percentage. Then, use that percentage to calculate your tax liability each week (This will be easy because there is a column for it on your revenue tracking spreadsheet). You can transfer this money from your business checking to your business savings. If you can't figure this out, contact an accountant to help you figure it out.

Make a checklist of regular weekly activities and create a new one each week. Wondering how you're going to remember to do all the right things each week and each of the tasks mentioned thus far? Don't worry; you'll have a Weekly Activities Checklist to keep you on track. You'll make a list of all the activities and use it to be sure you do what you need to before Saturday night. Each Sunday, after you write your weekly report, you'll print a new checklist for the coming week.

Write a weekly business report. List each day, what you did and what your goals are for the coming week. List any new business opportunities you closed. List your revenue generated and expenses. Write a few words on generally, how you felt about the week. It really doesn't matter if you send it anywhere; it's more about documenting what you did, setting goals and holding yourself accountable. If you can convince a mentor to review it weekly, even better. I am heading into my 4th year of business and have written one every week. I send it to my parents for their review.

Get your Linked In Profile up to date. Linked In is a business website, where Facebook is for social networking. While it's great to have both active, make sure your profile there is up to date. Ask friends to give you recommendations. Include all your professional jobs, not just yoga teaching jobs. Update your overall Summary section so it accurately reflects your passion, focus and what your business offers.

Create a one-page profile that includes all your experience, not just your teaching experience. Some yoga teachers that have corporate backgrounds wonder if it's helpful to include that on a resume that you might pass to a yoga studio or other teaching opportunity. The answer is a resounding "yes!" Everything you've done contributes to your value to any business. (More on this topic will be presented in the chapter on Resume Creation and Marketing).

Make sure you have teaching insurance. This becomes so important to protect you and your assets from any potential lawsuit. In addition, create a waiver to use when you teach outside a studio or do private sessions (sample included in this book).

Investigate what kind of business structure you want to have. Meet with an attorney and decide what kind of business structure you want and the implications for your taxes and tracking revenue and expenses.

Closing Summary

Building the infrastructure for your business requires the same discipline that a healthy yoga practice does; attention to detail, presence and flexibility. The time you spend setting up the processes and procedures for your day-to-day work will not only free you up to teach with a more relaxed, present style but it will help you ensure that you're growing your business and reaching the milestones you've set for yourself.

Chapter 5

Resume Creation and Marketing Your Classes

Focus

This chapter will provide guidelines for presenting professional work experience, yoga training, and teaching experience in resume format. A description of how to create a short biographical profile will also be provided for use on social media sites and on studio and other business websites. We will also review how to market classes and workshops via flyers, descriptions on studio websites and social media sites.

Overall Considerations

As big as the yoga industry is from a revenue and infrastructure perspective, with studios, teachers, magazines, products of all kinds, teacher training programs and workshops to cover every possible angle, it doesn't work much like any other industry when it comes to finding a job. Take a look at any studio website and there's no link for "Apply for Employment Here." A search for "yoga teaching jobs" on the Internet or job boards may pull up few leads in non-studio locations but you won't find much that's studio-based. Furthermore, many teachers decide they wish to teach yoga after years of working in a non-related industry so they're not sure how to present that information to prospective yoga-related employers.

As a result, for the new teacher who has invested time and money in training and is now done, there is often hesitancy around how to present a cohesive package to an employer and what to include. Also, because the yoga industry works very much on a "who you know" basis, many teachers never take the time to put a resume together and simply go with a profile or "bio" that's posted on studio websites once they've been hired. Also, as there are many yoga teachers in the industry, it's often difficult as a new teacher to differentiate yourself from other teachers, as a way to create a unique identity and leverage that uniqueness as a way to increase your chances of being hired.

While the related chapter to this one, called "Identifying and Evaluating Yoga Teaching Opportunities" will go into more detail about how to find job leads and evaluating them, this chapter will focus on creating the tools you need to put your best foot forward and also save time by having these tools available at all times. It will also help you differentiate yourself from others in the industry because so many teachers don't take the time to put a resume together.

Self-Evaluation

Start with an exploration about what you love about yoga and what led you to teaching

One of the best places to start when it comes to identifying your marketability (and therefore, "hire-ability") as a yoga teacher is with a description of what you love about yoga. Having this clear in your mind and expressed through a few short, clear statements will bring an authentic nature to your job search tools. While your resume won't necessarily have a section for "why you love yoga," it's important to have this clear in your mind for when you are asked by students and prospective employers for information about why you got into the industry in the first place.

Many teachers will say, "Yoga changed my life." While this may be true, it's helpful for the listener to have an idea of "how." Especially if your love of yoga comes from this kind of place, it's critical to the listener that they have more than this somewhat mysterious statement.

Think about it this way: if you meet someone on the street and they tell you they're thinking of going to their first yoga class but they're afraid to go for fear of being a beginner and they ask you, "Why did you get into yoga in the first place? What do you love about it?" What would you say?

Take a minute to answer that question

Then go back to your written statement and say it out loud. If it's more than 3 minutes, cut it down. Make it like an elevator pitch. Also, notice the words you're using to describe your feelings; if they're mystical, spiritual or hard to understand by someone that's unfamiliar with the yoga world, make it more relatable. While you want it to be authentic to you, you want it to also be clear to anyone that hears it.

Evaluate how your previous work experience makes you unique and skillful as a teacher

Depending on your previous non-yoga work experience, it may or may not be clear as to how it applies to your new career choice as a yoga teacher. If you worked in the medical field as a nurse or physician, perhaps that's more clear in terms of transferable skills you can use as a yoga teacher. Also, if you've worked in another wellness industry, such as a personal trainer or an exercise instructor of another kind, you may have an easier time illustrating how your past job will help you in your new role as yoga teacher.

However, just because your past job role isn't in the wellness or medical industry, doesn't mean you don't have transferable skills you'll use as a yoga teacher. Many people come to yoga after having management experience or other roles where they're responsible for managing teams of people. In these roles, they had to know how to motivate a group, keep a team moving forward towards a common goal and address individual performance in a way that supports growth on the individual level. This is not unlike the role you play as a yoga teacher when you're leading a group class.

Past work experience that includes speaking to groups, working as part of a team, being creative, being expressive, thinking on your feet, managing in situations where things can change at a moment's notice all provide great experience for the role of yoga teacher. For many new teachers, updating their current resume with yoga teaching information may be the way to go because there is so much relevant non-teaching experience.

Take a few minutes and outline what past work experiences you can apply to your teaching and why.

Evaluate how your personal experiences make you unique and skillful as a yoga teacher

Almost more than any other job, being an inspiring and well-rounded yoga teacher means that you'll be using much more than the techniques you learned in teacher training when you step into the classroom. If you only used that information, your classes may come across as flat and one-dimensional. But when you connect to who you are and what make you a unique individual and learn how to have the courage to show that to your students, rather than standing behind some idea of "what a yoga teacher should be like," you will find your unique voice as a teacher.

For instance, there are many yoga teachers that are also parents. Being a parent is a challenging and rewarding job at the same time. There is much that as parents, people have to do in order to inspire and guide their children. While yoga teachers don't want to be "parenting" their students, a newer teacher who is also a parent has their own strengths in that role that can be useful in bringing to their teaching.

The same would be true for someone who has overcome some kind of personal struggle in order to get where they are in life. Whether it's due to some physical or emotional battle, overcoming this kind of obstacle can give you wonderful content for your resume and also for your teaching. It also can make you stand out as a teacher and help you start to build your own unique identity.

Take a few minutes and think of the personal experiences you've had and how they might enrich your yoga teaching.

Determine what your ideal vision is for your yoga teaching

Just as in any other job market, you need to have an understanding of what you want to do and the kinds of job you want to have, so you can state it clearly both in writing and when someone you meets asks you. Just like in your "Why I love Yoga" statement, this vision will help you as you go out and evaluate opportunities and will help friends and colleagues understand what you're looking to do.

Write down what your ideal vision is for your yoga teaching.

Identify who your target audience is for your teaching

There are so many options for teaching yoga and many exist outside the traditional studio environment. Adults, children of varying ages, families, seniors, athletes of all kinds and expectant mothers are just some of people who might enjoy your classes. Part of helping you find a job and create a powerful resume includes an understanding of the group you wish to teach.

Who do you wish to teach?

Resume and Bio Creation

For the focus on writing your resume, we'll focus on what should be different on your professional teaching resume from just general business resumes. For the purposes of our conversation, it's assumed you'll use the formatting you wish and include your name, address and contact phone. However, here are some additional tips to consider when creating a professional teaching resume:

About teaching and training experience:

- Start with a statement as to the kind of yoga opportunities you are interesting in pursuing ("I'm interested in working with children, families and teaching pre-natal yoga")
- If you have a yoga website, include it
- If you have an email that is attached to that website, include that as your contact email, not your regular email address
- It is up to you if you wish to blend in your professional business experience with your yoga teaching experience so items appear in chronological order or, if you prefer, you can put your teaching and training experience at the top of the resume and the professional experience at the bottom
- Include the name and dates of attendance for your major teaching training program
- Include the level of Yoga Alliance registration you carry and the date associated with that designation
- Include a statement about the style of yoga you teach
- If you carry a separate certification from the yoga school that you attended, include that as well

- List the studios and other locations for which you currently teach, include dates of hire and number of classes
- Resist listing every workshop you attended. Stick with the major events/trainings
- If you have conducted workshops, include dates and locations, or if many, include a general statement indicating the kinds of trainings you have held
- If you have assisted a mentor/more senior teacher, worked as an apprentice, been a general assistant at a studio or worked as a volunteer at a studio, include this
- If you are CPR and First Aid certified (which you should be) include this and date of award
- If you have any other related training, include it.

About your professional experience:

- Include your corporate/business jobs with Job role, dates, name of employer
- Only include a brief statement regarding overall job role
- Focus on job skills that are transferable to yoga teaching ("led team meetings, managed team of 15 developers, created and presented to corporate management.")

About your educational experience:

This can be a standard section, as in regular resumes, including schools, diplomas and dates.

About you/Other Highlights:

Include any brief comments or bullets about things/activities/achievements unique to you. These items might come from one of the above sections on experiences that make you unique, such as completing a marathon, writing for a wellness publication or volunteering.

Creating your Bio Statement:

Once you start teaching at studios, they will request a picture (have one you like ready to go that shows your face clearly, rather than you in a complicated yoga pose) and a short statement about you for posting on their website. Having this ready to email quickly will allow you to complete this request easily and will endear you to studio owners and business managers who may need to chase people down to get this information. Your biographical paragraph is what the students will see when they "check you out" on the website so tailor it to them. Include things such as:

- Your teaching style/Certification/Registration/Training school
- Why you love yoga and what inspires you about teaching (as in above exercise)
- A short statement as to what your students can expect in your classes
- Your contact information/website.

Refrain from using highly technical words, Sanskrit and artistic descriptions. These will only confuse students. Keep it basic and informative. Let the more spiritual and creative aspect of your teaching come out in class.

Marketing Classes and Workshops

The marketing of classes and workshops is mainly done via the Internet on websites of the studios and locations at which you will be teaching.

For studio classes:

Make sure YOU write the description of YOUR class. Use clear and generally understandable language (refrain from a great deal of Sanskrit and other yoga related words and phrasing, unless you provide the English translation). Tell the reader what to expect (time, length of class, if props are used, general style of class) and also indicate if the class is appropriate for all levels of students.

This description will be on the website of any location at which you teach.

For workshops:

Include the date, time, location and cost. If there is a discount for early registration, include it. If students need to bring any special clothing, writing materials or equipment, include it in the description. Again, use language that's clear and understandable for anyone, regardless of yoga experience or previous exposure. A description of your workshop will go on the website of the location at which you're teaching.

If you use a personal and/or business Facebook page and/or Twitter, write a brief notice about it there and post a reminder about it a few times a week. You can also create a specific invitation for the event. If you have a blog on your website, write a post about what people can expect if they attend.

Make a flyer for the studio door and inside the studio. Ask the studio owner if there is a format he/she prefers and keep it as a template for future use.

If the community has a local paper and/or community website, include a post about it there if you can.

Look for business groups, community groups and other networking groups that might be interested in your topic and let them know about your event. If your event is a children's yoga class, let the local Mother's Association know about it. If there are other exercise facilities in the neighborhood (that don't offer yoga) let them know about it as they may wish to do some cross marketing. Offer them a stipend if they refer students to your workshop.

Tell your friends, neighbors and any local family members.

Closing Summary

Having these tools on hand and ready will allow you to move efficiently through your day because you'll have these things when requested by potential employers. You'll also distinguish yourself from other teachers by having a well thought out resume and bio ready to go.

Chapter 6

Identifying and Evaluating Yoga Teaching Opportunities and Pricing Your Class

Focus

This chapter will provide guidelines for seeking out yoga teaching jobs. It will provide information on finding jobs, evaluate the nature of opportunities from a variety of perspectives (not just rate of pay) and will provide other avenues for teaching yoga outside of the traditional "in-studio" teaching jobs.

Overall Considerations

When yoga teachers graduate from a training program, while they are armed with the technical skills to teach a yoga class, they are often without an understanding around how to find a teaching job. Unlike other industries, the yoga community has not (yet) established much of the same job-seeking infrastructure that many other (most other) industries have. That is to say, studios rarely, if ever, have a job seeking page on their website, there aren't head hunters or recruiters that assist a teacher in finding a job, and many yoga jobs are not posted on job boards or other generally used job seeker websites. As a result, new teachers are left to develop a network for the purpose of finding a job. Many times, teachers will contact a studio, only to hear, "We only hire teachers that graduate from our own teacher training program." This can be discouraging and can lead to feelings of confusion and resentment and even jealously towards teachers that do teach in these studios.

Also, teachers that graduate from specialty programs or those that wish to focus their teaching in certain areas, besides adult classes, face a bigger challenge because they most likely won't be teaching in a general studio. The teacher that wishes to teach outside of a studio needs to work even harder to generate leads and opportunities to teach and in many cases, may be the first person to be contacting a location regarding teaching yoga.

For the new yoga teacher, the most important thing is to start teaching immediately. The longer one waits after graduating, the harder it is to start teaching because usually the biggest resistance to teaching is fear. The longer one thinks about it, the fear element creates a barrier. Therefore, it is helpful to start developing your network and leads before you graduate from training so you can transition into a teaching job right after you're done.

Strategy

Here are some general tips to start your job search process:

Start with your yoga teacher-training program. The yoga community is based on interpersonal connections and even more so, since there is very little (as mentioned above) established in terms of formal job search process. Before you graduate (and, I'd even suggest you include this as part of the process to evaluate a potential yoga training program) ask the lead teacher how the program will provide you with help in finding a job. If the program is hosted at a particular studio, find out what opportunities exist to teach there. If there are opportunities to volunteer your time at the studio where you did training, or be an assistant in class, do it. Even those jobs that are non-paying are great ways to develop relationships and be available when new opportunities arise.

Contact studios near your home. One of the biggest challenges for yoga teachers is getting from class to class. The more you can decrease your travel time, the more teaching you can do with less stress and loss of income. Find yoga studios that are nearby and contact them direct (more on how to do this later). The fact that you're close by will be an advantage to them as well.

Develop a network of teachers. Start with your fellow graduates from teacher training. Add in mentors you regularly contact and from whom you take class. Include the names of studio owners you contact. Maintain their information in your Business Dashboard. Look on the website of your teacher training school and find other graduates of the program. Use Facebook to find other teachers that teach your style of yoga. Include all these names in your database and use them to contact for job leads.

Use Craig's list and Indeed.com to find posted jobs. Yoga studios, while they do not have a job opportunity page on their website, may post teaching jobs on Craig's list. Also, non-studio teaching jobs may be found on other sites (for instance, corporate wellness jobs or jobs in other non-studio locations). Indeed.com is a job site that pulls jobs from many websites so the job seeker doesn't need to individually gather leads from each major site.

Contact teachers that are currently on staff at local studios to find out how they were hired. It never hurts to ask someone how they got a teaching job and in the process, you might make a connection to a new teacher you can add to your network.

Ask to be on the substitute list of local studios. Studios are always looking for substitutes and many have lists of teachers they can call on when they are in a bind. When you contact studios, if they tell you they are not hiring, ask if you can be on their substitute list.

Attend workshops. Now that you're done with teacher training, it's easy to think that the learning stops. Nothing could be further from the truth. Keep your eye open for one-day workshops at local studios to keep yourself in learning mode. This is also a great way to network with teachers, because many attend workshops.

Become a saavy Facebook ,Twitter and Instagram user. Social networking has changed the way we meet people, make business connections, share ideas and further the relationships we already have. For those that are naysayers about the time wasting aspect of social networking, they're using it to waste time on the application. As a new yoga teacher, connect to as many fellow teachers as possible. Look for what they are doing. Connect to studios. Post information about what you're looking for and what you're interested in doing from a specialty perspective. Answer any email you get promptly and in a friendly manner. Be professional! Write every post with a sense that it would be safe for ANYONE to read. It is a great source of networking.

Offer your services for free. Look for opportunities to offer free classes at worksites, friend's homes, parties, wellness conferences, road races and other community events. Anything you do is an opportunity to make a connection and be seen as a wellness expert in the field of yoga.

Locating specific non-studio teaching jobs

If you're interested in teaching outside a studio setting, it can be daunting to try to identify where you might teach. Here are some ideas for locations that may be interested in having a yoga teacher visit to offer classes. Remember, one of the advantages to teaching in these settings is you will be the only one negotiating the details of your class and your class may be the only class offered. This often can help you negotiate a higher rate of pay and you can be a resource for general wellness rather than only be accessed for teaching classes.

Schools: Pre-schools, grade schools, high schools and colleges are all options. Kids of all ages need yoga; they're more stressed than ever and overwhelmed with life. Secondly, it's hard to find a common time to offer a class in a neighborhood and get good turnout. Once you bring the yoga to them, you don't have to worry about scheduling; they're already there. Talk to the principal or director and make your pitch.

Non-Profits: There are many non-profits that serve children. The Boys and Girls Club, Big Brothers Big Sisters and the Girls and Boy Scouts are some common ones. If you have a personal or professional relationship with a Non Profit, ask them if you can serve their population by providing yoga. In some cases, you'll be doing it for free but think of it as good karma as well as a valuable relationship to nurture. You'll be serving a worthy population and there are many influential community leaders associated with the Boards of Directors of non-profits. You'll be able to develop good connections through your yoga teaching there.

Sport Organizations: Think about groups in your area that serve athletes of all kinds. Running clubs, non-profits that serve rowers, walking clubs, sports clubs, ski clubs; basically any sports group that hosts sporting activities might find yoga useful before or after their events.

Mothers Associations/ Women's Clubs: Women are more stressed than ever these days as many balance their own needs with those of their families. They're ripe for wanting to do something healthy but hard-pressed to find a way to squeeze in the time. If your neighborhood has a Mother's Association, meet with the group's leader. Women's Clubs may meet in your neighborhood; see if you can attend a meeting to do a demonstration. If they're interested, you can consider holding regular classes at their meetings or off-site.

Homes for seniors/ Assisted Living Centers: What better place to share yoga than with seniors? They'll love the conversation, doing something different, connecting with their breath and you'll love their smiles as they try out the poses.

Golf Clubs: Learning how to firmly root into your feet, rotating your torso while keeping your hips centered, coordinating breathing with movement; these are some of the keys of golf which yoga can provide. Create a proposal about yoga for golfers and send it out to a few clubs. If you have a personal contact with a member, that will come in handy too.

Local Parks: Organizations in your neighborhood may host events at your local parks. Here in Boston, The Esplanade Association hosts everything from the Boston Pops Fourth of July event to outdoor exercise classes. Contact your local groups about hosting yoga outdoors. They'll help you get the permits you need to run your classes.

Local businesses: Talk to businesses in your area. Check out any local lists of "Top Employers in your Area." Top employers, as voted on by employees, value health and wellness and offer in-house services. These are great employers to go to regarding onsite yoga. Think of unique ways to bring yoga into the workplace besides traditional classes; yoga-at-your-desk, guided meditation and classes that focus on tight hips might be a place to start.

Physical Therapy offices: More and more therapists are referring their patients to yoga. Connect with some to see if they have an interest in some in-house yoga. You'll learn a ton about the body and you can both collaborate on treatment plans for clients.

Holistic Wellness Centers: Similar to therapy offices, check out local wellness centers. These may be community centers, space that houses a team of chiropractors, acupuncturists and massage therapists. Yoga would be a great addition to their team.

How to contact a studio or other location regarding teaching classes

As with all things, it's always better to contact someone if you have a mutual connection. If you share a friend or business contact, mention them when you reach out via email. If you can contact the studio owner via email, that's usually a good start because studio owners have variable schedules and are hard to catch via the phone that rings in the studio. If you have a yoga resume, include that with the email.

You can contact a studio owner or manager via the email address on their website. Someone that works for the owner usually manages it. Keep the email professional and appropriate to be read by anyone. Also, remember that studio owners are in and out of the studio and there may be a lag time from when you leave the message to it reaching them. Give them time to respond before you try contacting them again if you have not heard.

If they are on Facebook, send them a message via Facebook asking them only what the best way is for reaching them. Many people prefer to get work related emails via their work email address, so a simple message asking for the best way to connect with them will suffice.

When you connect with the owner, let them know you are interested in teaching classes. Give them an opportunity to say if they are looking for teachers. Be ready to send your resume if you haven't already and be ready with your 3 minute pitch statement that highlights your training, experience and the style of yoga you teach.

Some studios will only hire teachers that have completed their teacher training program, so don't be discouraged if you get this as feedback. Some managers will request you come for an audition, so be prepared.

SPECIAL NOTE: When doing any audition, KEEP THE SEQUENCING SIMPLE. Auditions are not the time for you to show off your latest "yoga challenge" pose or to show off your most creative sequence. You'll be nervous, which is natural. The worst thing you can do is select a complex sequence. YOU want to shine through and have space for expression and to inspire; this is very hard if you are throwing out lots of instruction around the poses. Unless the person requesting the audition specifically selects you to do a specific thing, stick with Sun Salutations or something very basic.

Contacting other job opportunities outside of studios is a bit different. The above list of non-studio teaching locations presents a bit about strategies around contacting them. As a general rule, have a brief pitch, look for a common thread you can use to build a connection (if you have had contact with the organization or you know someone there, or you use their services or product or you just read about them in the news- these are all great to mention). Keep track of all of these leads in your Business Dashboard and follow up like mad to see them through a resolution (either closed deal or not).

Negotiating a rate for your classes

Many studios will have a set rate for teachers. This means that there may be very little you can do in the way of negotiating. This can be challenging also if you're new and don't have much experience. If this is the case, you need to decide if the teaching job is worth it from other perspectives outside of revenue (see the section on "Evaluating a Teaching Opportunity"). Some studio owners will be open to negotiating a rate and/or the basis of the rate (flat rate or variable, depending on number of students in class).

You also need to have a sense of your worth as a teacher, which in part, is determined by your experience. Experience is worth more to studio owners because it shows that you have been in the trenches and are able to handle a wider variety of students. The kind of training you have, depth of training, hours of training and the recognition of your teacher training program to the studio owner may all be part of what you consider to be part of your worth as a teacher.

You also need to have an idea of what the local market is bearing as reimbursement rates for yoga teachers. This data is a little harder to get because there's no database that will show you rates for yoga teachers. You can try to ask teachers you know for a range rather than asking them, "What do you get paid?" but you may or may not get the answers. Generally speaking, teachers are paid between $30 and $75 a class but this is a very general range and may not apply to teaching in non-studio locations and to teachers who have more experience.

Before you contact the studio owner, know the rate you want. Know the leeway (up or down, although 'down' is usually the only one you'll need to be concerned with) on which you're willing to concede. If it ends up that you can't agree on terms but it still is a good opportunity or connection, ask if you can be on their substitute list. If not, keep them in mind for the future. You never know in the future, if things change, they may reach out to you.

Be sure with any teaching job that you clarify BEFORE you start how and when you will be paid. Some questions to clarify:

- How will you be paid? Check, cash or other form of payment (i.e. Pay Pal)
- When will you be paid?
- Will taxes be taken out of your pay?
- Do you need to submit an invoice? If so, when?
- Do you need to fill out a W4?
- Do you need to fill out any other paperwork in order to get into their payroll system?
- If checks are not mailed, how will you receive them?

Evaluating a teaching opportunity

When looking for teaching jobs, there are many factors to use to evaluate the position. One of the most obvious and tangible factors is rate of pay. What you'll be paid is a valid concern and one that factors into the relationship with any employer. However, there are many other factors as well and in fact, some of the most valuable relationships you may have are with those for whom you teach for free. Free events can give you broad exposure to a wide audience, can introduce you to people that don't usually practice yoga (because the "free" angle makes it really attractive), can often connect you to strategic contacts (as the events are often hosted by non-profit foundations, wellness organizations or other influential resources) and have the added benefit of bringing you the good karma that comes with doing something for free.

Some of the other factors that should be considered when looking at a teaching job:

- Distance from your home and/or travel needed
- Time of class
- Opportunity for other business to be developed (workshops, teacher trainings)
- The opportunity to help you spread the word about your teaching due to their large reach
- The opportunity to be part of a larger teaching community that is related to your training; i.e. the studio is one of the locations that hosts the training you completed
- The opportunity allows you to teach a specialty kind of yoga or to a specialty group; i.e. yoga for athletes, for children or pre-natal yogaThe opportunity meets one of your business objectives; i.e. you want to teach children as part of your yoga offeringYou need the money
- You need to start teaching

Closing Summary

Due to the widespread appeal of yoga in our culture, the opportunities for teaching yoga are multiple and varied. However, with the proliferation of teacher training programs, there are many teachers out there too. The more you can hone in on what you want to do, the types of locations in which you want to teach and what your value-add is to an employer, the more successful you'll be in closing yoga teaching jobs.

As with everything, do your homework, pay attention to the details, keep all your correspondence professional and follow up like mad.

Chapter 7

Making the Switch from Corporate Work to Teaching Yoga

Focus

Many people begin a yoga practice after working for many years in the traditional corporate environment. When they graduate from a training program, there are often many questions about how to make the switch to a teaching job. The objective of this chapter is to provide you with several factors to consider before making the switch.

Overall Considerations

The yoga industry is filled with teachers that have varied background and experience from a variety of sources. While the lineage and training of the forefathers of yoga was based on practicing and teaching from a young age, teachers today often transition to yoga teaching from working in the corporate world or for a business, organization or other full-time employment. Upon completion of a training program, many teachers feel the urge, or actually do, quit their regular full-time position, as they're energized and inspired about the possibilities of teaching yoga full-time. In many cases, this can leave people with debt, frustration and regret as they realize that they cannot bring in enough money to cover their basic expenses. What I'm going to suggest below will take time and surely isn't as fun as buying yoga clothes or taking class or just sticking your head in the sand and quitting your job, hoping it all works. Take it from my experience of living through a significant level of debt built up over 3 years; the time you spend now will save you financial hardship and much frustration in the future.

With some planning and preparation, there are ways to transition from full-time employment outside the yoga industry to a full-time role as a yoga teacher. What we'll cover below are the factors to consider in order to give yourself the best opportunity for success.

Strategy

The first step is to evaluate and "check yourself" around the idea of teaching yoga full-time. You may think you want to do it but are you romanticizing the idea of teaching yoga based on your perception of what the lifestyle is like? There are certain factors to consider when thinking about teaching full-time:

1. Decide if you're an independent worker or if you prefer the structure of a company. Even yoga teachers that work for one studio system or own their own studio are essentially, entrepreneurs. Outside of teaching classes, your non-teaching time will be consumed by doing your own marketing, budgeting, planning and new business development. If these aren't your strong suits, there may not be anyone else to lean on (unless you get a business partner that has these skills). Before you jump ship on your corporate job, be honest with yourself about your skills and what you really like to do.

2. Decide on the full-time teaching model you most would like to pursue. You may decide you'd like the "brick and mortar" model of owning a studio. You might like to fully commit to one studio system and teach all your classes there. You might decide to start your own brand and teach in a variety of studios and other locations. There are many different forms a yoga teaching job can take and it's helpful to know what you'd most prefer.

3. Talk to teachers that are already living the life. I remember after my first teacher training with Baron Baptiste, being in the airport on the way home to Boston. I was with one of the teachers that led the training and she was going through her appointment book. At the time, I was working full time and I'd just had the most amazing experience in training. I remember thinking: "I want her life!" Honestly, I had little detail about what her life was like outside of my own perceptions. After that, I spent months talking to teachers about lifestyle, schedule, finances, challenges, rewards and all aspects of teaching. It was helpful to ask them about both the pitfalls and highlights of the career.

4. Decide if certification is important to you. Many teachers from whom you'll pursue training have their own certification process. Some of these programs will be recognized by Yoga Alliance and some will not. As discussed in an earlier chapter, part of your preparation to either work for one of these teachers in their studios or working for yourself is to determine if you think it's important/necessary/helpful to be "Certified" by the teacher from whom you receive training (You may also be required to get Certified by a particular teacher if you want to teach for them in their studios). This can be a costly process but can also be one that provides you with an affiliation to a larger organization. This may be helpful from a marketing and teaching opportunity perspective as well as connecting you to a community of like-minded teachers. It can also give the yoga students you meet a way to connect you to a particular style and training process. Decide if you think this is important to have and if so, select training programs that will provide you with the certification and registration status from Yoga Alliance that you would ultimately like.

5. Get down to brass tacks about money (more on this below). As with any potential job switch, it's always helpful to look at the financial aspects. Start with what you know (your expenses). If you don't have a monthly budget, make one now and figure out the bare minimum you need to break even (I included a sample for you). Then, with that number in mind, start to map out the opportunities you'd need to generate that income. Not sure how much you'll be paid? Ask other teachers about it. Within reason, teachers can give you a range of rates for different services (group classes, privates, freelance work). See what you'd need to generate on your own in order to hit your number.

6. Don't rule out teaching part-time first. If you're in the process of this analysis and not getting the results you want, don't rule out the idea of teaching part-time while working. This allows you to start out while having the support of a corporate salary and benefits.

7. Consider the importance of health insurance, retirement savings and taxes. Most yoga teachers get health insurance on their own, as it's not provided by their employer(s). Teachers that transi-

tioned to teaching full-time after using company sponsored 401K plans may have either kept those funds in the 401K or moved them to an IRA. In either event, your retirement savings is most often up to you to do, if this is important to you. Also, many yoga teachers need to do their own taxes as well as make estimated payments throughout the year. You may want to consider hiring an accountant to help you plan for the year ahead.

Once you've done an honest evaluation and have decided that your intention is to teach yoga full-time, the next step is to do a financial review so you can determine how much money you'll need to make to:

- Cover monthly expenses, including health and teaching insurance
- Leave yourself enough money for some living expenses each month

The reason you want to do this now is because the worst case scenario is one where you quit your full-time job and realize you can't secure enough teaching jobs to cover your expenses, let alone leave you any spending money. The best case scenario is that you take the time to do an evaluation of not only your expenses but the number of classes and other teaching gigs you'd need to book and then start to work to secure these before you leave your job (this also gives you time to start to save money to hold you over or get a part-time job as a way to be earning some money while you are starting to teach).

Begin with your budget. I've included a form you can use as a start. You'll customize this form by adding in items that are relevant to you. Remember, these are your fixed costs every month. These things may change by a few dollars (things like cell phone, heat, gas) but they appear monthly. Other fixed costs that don't change are items like rent or mortgage, any condo fees or insurance for the car and home.

Savings should be one of your first priorities, even before your bills. Paying yourself for the work you do is just as important as paying your creditors. For now, take a monthly amount and budget it into your fixed costs on your budget worksheet. This amount may change but for now, pick a number so you have something budgeted. Once you have this annual number, break it down into a monthly, weekly and then daily number, using the number of days you wish to work per week. For teachers, remember that 1- you need a day off and 2-even if you work 6 days a week, you may have a few hours each day where you are not working so it may be manageable. This daily number becomes the amount of money you need to earn each day in order to make your annual salary number.

Create the Business Dashboard (discussed in the chapter on "Building Your Yoga-Preneurship"). At the top, put your desired annual salary. Include the monthly, weekly and daily breakdown so you end up with your daily number identified at the top. Then create sections. One section is "Studio classes." One section might be "Corporate classes." One might be " Wellness Presentations." One might be "Senior Yoga." One might be "Children's Services." Then enter the work you currently have in black text (if any- because remember, starting your teaching part-time is a great, low risk way to get into teaching). Include the rate and multiply by the number of times in a month you teach that class and enter your monthly revenue. Add up the numbers and see what you get as your monthly salary and multiply by 12. This is the actual annual salary you are currently earning (gross).

Adjust to meet your financial goal number. Chances are, the annual figure is less than your desired annual salary (if it's not, good for you!) This is a common experience. Many teachers are living well below their salary requirements, which is why they build up credit card debt and "go without." So, now, go back to your spreadsheet, and in red, add teaching opportunities to each section. Keep adding until you get to the total monthly revenue that allows you to meet your annual number. Think out of the box! If you don't, you'll always be working short of your goal. If you think, "I'll never be able to get 3 corporate teaching gigs per month," you're right, you never will. But if you identify it as a job that helps you reach your overall goal, you will be able to take directed action on the marketing side of your activities to seek out opportunities that help you meet your financial goals. This discussion will pertain more to the independent yoga teacher versus the studio owner, as that's a very different business model. However, to a certain extent, the steps above still pertain to a studio owner. You need to know how much money you need to make each month to cover your expenses; whether that money comes from teaching classes or people that work for you teaching classes.

Set your rates for service. One thing that you need to consider that is a piece of this analysis is: what will you charge per service? Well, now that you've figured out what you have to earn each day in order to make your annual salary, you'll have an idea of what your rate might be. This does not mean that you'll charge $200 for a private, just to help you work less and meet your goal. Let's say your daily number is $200 and you've assumed you'll work 6 days a week. Using $50 per studio class as a rate (this is just a number I selected for this exercise), you'd need to teach 4 studio classes per DAY in order to reach your number. While you may think you can physically do this (which may not be realistic), the reality of finding 4 classes per day to teach in your area may be slim. So, you can see you need to have a "blend" of teaching opportunities, with different rates, in order to make things work. You need to also consider what others are charging (ask other teachers), the complexity of the teaching gig (custom sequences, working with specialty groups, like children for instance), the travel involved, if you need to take any special training, the time involved from start to finish for the gig (travel included), your level of experience and any other factor that pertains to you and the job. This list of rates should cover anything that you've listed as a teaching activity (actual or desired).

Now that you've done the analysis to determine one approach to teaching that will cover your expenses, do you still want to leave your full-time job? As I mentioned before, you may want to start out teaching part-time. If you think teaching yoga part-time is a cop-out on your dream, think about these reasons to try it first:

Financial: When you're teaching yoga part time, you usually (might not) have to depend on the income. This can free you up to teach where you want, when you want, without any sense of having to fill your schedule with the first opportunities that arise. You also will have more stability in your financial life so you can continue to meet your obligations.

A chance to gain experience: Teaching yoga part time can give you the time to gain some experience before (and if) you choose to teach full time. When you're just starting out, you may feel like while you learned the mechanics of teaching in training, you are still trying to manage the classroom and all that goes along with that. While you teach part time, you can still attend trainings, read, meet with other teachers and luxuriate in the joys of learning something new.

Less impact from fluctuations in your teaching schedule: As a yoga teacher, sometimes things shift in your schedule when you least expect it. This may not be a reflection on you, but may be for reasons completely out of your control. If you teach in a studio, there may be changes in the schedule that affect your classes. If you're teaching in a school, the classes may end when the school year ends. If you're teaching private students, sessions can be canceled for illness or travel. This is why it's critical to have a pipeline of opportunities and always be networking so you can try to fill in openings as they arise. When you're teaching part time, you've got a little insulation from these variations.

Health Insurance: One of the practical considerations when teaching full time is health insurance. As a teacher, you will most likely not receive health insurance from any of the employers you work with so if you're not on someone else's policy, you'll need to get it for yourself (if you indeed want health insurance). Teaching part time will allow you to maintain your coverage.

A chance to "try-on" teaching to see if it's a lifestyle for you: Making the shift from working full time in a corporate-type job to working independently as a yoga teacher can be big change. Finding teaching gigs, figuring out how best to spend your non-teaching time, managing the administrative aspects, including taxes, marketing, scheduling, correspondence and program development may not be your strong suits. In your part time role, you can start to manage these things a little bit and see how you do.

A way to feed your dharma while you're in the corporate world: If you feel that teaching yoga is your true calling, then you'll be doing yourself a huge disservice by denying yourself a chance to try it out. Also, if you're frustrated in your regular job, one of the best ways to shift from that negativity is to do something you love. Feeding your true passion will allow you to head into your regular job feeling like you're investing in yourself too; not just giving away all your energy to something you don't love.

If you've gone through the above analysis and you've decided that full-time and only full-time independent teaching will do, here are some action steps you can take to make the shift:

Start to market yourself as a teacher. See if you can secure some jobs part time as a transition to teaching full-time.

Start connecting with studios and discuss their hiring policy. Meet with studio owners, email for information and network with other teachers you know. Find out more about how teachers on the schedule are hired. See if you can audition for a regular class slot or at least a slot as a substitute.

Start saving money from your regular job. You will need to build up a nest egg that can help carry you over from your salary to your teaching salary.

Find a health insurance provider and set up a date to transfer to a new carrier. This will mean you have to select a date to make the switch. I won't go into all the reasons why having health insurance is critical again; I've covered it before. To choose to leave a job and not make arrangements for other coverage is just plain risky. The financial ruin you could put yourself in should you get ill and not have coverage is significant. In order to protect yourself from a break in coverage, you need to switch from one carrier to the next. This is why selecting a new carrier is important to do before quitting your current job.

Get teaching insurance. This is for your protection and helps to ensure that you are protected in the event of a claim.

Take on some weeknight and weekend classes. This will give you a chance to build your network, start teaching and get on the substitute list for the studios in which you teach. This will also start you on the path to earning money. All this new earned income should go into a savings account. This is going to be the nest egg you live off of until your teaching income is where you need it to be to cover your expenses. This is also the account into which you will make deposits from your corporate job. Save as much as you can! I actually sold my house and bought a condo and used the profit to jumpstart my savings account. Think about the kind of lifestyle you want as a yoga teacher. For me, it was more important for me to be in Boston and close to the studio I was teaching in at the time than to be in a bigger place that required a longer drive.

Decide on a breaking point where you will make the switch. Decide how much money you need in your savings account before you switch. Remember, depending on your financial needs and the rate at which you can save, it might be several months. This is where the rubber meets the road. You can leave your corporate job too soon and you'll end up in debt. You can do what's necessary to save money and make the switch when you have the money saved. This is always the better approach and will save you much heartache in the long run. When to make the switch may also be a function of if you have someone else helping you out financially, like a significant other or family.

Pick your day and celebrate! Once you decide on the switch day, make sure all the loose ends in your corporate job are tied up neatly. Remember, nothing is final! You never know when you may need those contacts. In fact, your corporate job may be a great opportunity to teach corporate yoga! Take yourself out to dinner and celebrate your planning, execution and the beginning of a new career doing what you love!

Closing Summary

Making any kind of career change is a big move. There are always risks but with solid planning, being truthful with yourself about your needs- both financial and otherwise- you can create a plan that, once executed, will set you up for success in your new job. Teaching yoga is in large part, a matter of the heart. But to do it right, it requires solid planning too.

Chapter 8

Using Your Website and Social Media to Create Brand Awareness

Focus

In the late 90's and early 2000's, teachers built a name for themselves by teaching classes. There was no Facebook, Twitter, Instagram, hashtags or Throwback Thursdays. There was just the need to show up, be there for your class and teach a solid flow. This was how you built your name and grew your classes. In today's world though, the methods we use to communicate have changed. It's much more electronically triggered and the yoga world is no different. Teachers don't have to, but it can be helpful to build a website and participate in social media not only as a way to let people know when you're teaching but also to build a network of clients, friends and colleagues.

Overall Considerations

As mentioned above, there are several aspects to building the electronic infrastructure to support your teaching. For certain, having an electronic presence will help you build your classes and the people that know about you and your brand, but having a following on social media is not a substitute for being skilled at providing quality in-person teaching. However, it is a commonly used practice to post on social media, direct people to your website for your schedule and use these electronic tools to build your brand. Let's take a look at some of the components of building your brand using your website and social media.

Make special note that we'll begin this discussion with a focus on your website. While some might think having a Facebook page should be the central component of your internet strategy, the reality is having a well-built website is critical and should be the central hub of your electronic "face." Why? Well, first of all, you design it (or someone you hire will), you update it, you can change it at will and unless you want it to, it will never be removed. Unlike Facebook, Twitter and other social media sites, you control the content and the rules of use for your visitors. The reality is these popular social media sites have increasingly made it harder and harder, especially for small business owners (like yoga teachers) to use their sites to build a following. Their main focus is on revenue generation once they've amassed a significant following. As a result, your posts won't be seen by as many people as you want unless you pay to have your posts viewed by more than a handful of your subscribers. Further, as people use more and more of these sites throughout the day, the chance that they will see your post decreases as well. And, lastly, as everyone is running short on time, the amount of time they spend online and actually "seeing" your posts… well, the probability of that goes down also.

So, what can you do? Well, you need to build two things: 1- a website, as mentioned before and 2- a mailing list. The mailing list will allow you to stay in touch with people who have chosen (note: we're not putting people on a mailing list; they are opting in) to stay in touch with you. Your mailing list, when used wisely, will allow you to create special emails to your mailing list subscribers. While email might seem antiquated when compared to the flashy pages of Facebook and Twitter, the reality is there is a much greater chance that one of your subscribers will see your email and open it, than will see your post on social media.

Building a website is a chapter all its own as is the task of building your mailing list but start with the premise that you'll build a solid website and with it, sign up for a mailing list service (I use MailChimp and really like it). Remember, you can always hire someone to build it for you as well. This person can work with you on specific tasks and teach you how to maintain your site and make simple changes. If you don't know anyone who has the skills to build a website, post your request on www.taskrabbit.com. Task Rabbit is an excellent resource to find high quality professionals to do tasks of all kinds.

Let's talk about some of the components of your website:

About you. This page will describe a bit about you, your background, your teaching experience and anything else that you wish to share. It should be professional but also should allow for people to get a sense of who you are.

Schedule. This should detail your public classes and include links to the studios, class times and a short description of the type of class (heated flow yoga, restorative, etc.)

Articles. If you have a regular writing gig someplace and write articles or if you've written articles in the past, have a page where you can link to them here. This will allow your website visitors to see your articles and find out about other areas of expertise that you have (all yoga related, of course)

Events. This should be a page that lists any special events (outside of classes) that you have. These could include workshops, trainings, children's classes, speaking engagements or free events.

Contact. This page should have a link to a "Contact Me" email that will allow a visitor to send you an email. You should have an email that is related to your website (karen@barebonesyoga.com is the email for my website, www.barebonesyoga.com)

There are other pages you can build as well. This is just a starter list.

The Mailing List:

Building a mailing list will give you a way to stay in touch with people who have decided they want to stay in touch with you. Much like a "fan" to your Facebook page or a "follower" on your Twitter or Instagram profile, these are people who have decided that they want to stay in touch with what you're doing. Just as with these social media sites, your mailing list is "opt in/opt out" which means that just as they can opt in to receive your notices, they can also opt out at any time when they decide that they no longer wish to stay in touch. So, the word to the wise is this: use your link to your mailing list subscribers judiciously! Only send emails when they are absolutely necessary. Also, if you decide to do things like send videos or newsletters, get into a regular pattern so people will come to depend on seeing them.

Here are some ways you can use your mailing list:

Create a newsletter: Use this to inform your subscribers of up and coming events and remind them of your schedule. If there are any chances to your schedule, highlight them here. Offer tips, articles and videos; remember, the newsletter should be more than a promotion. In fact, it must be informative if you wish to build credibility. As a result, use it to provide information more than promote. I use the same sections from week to week and simply switch out or update the content in each section. Also, decide how often you will send it out and stick to that schedule as much as possible. People will come to depend on your newsletter and hopefully share it with others.

Send out alerts about special events: Again, use this judiciously as you don't want to be a pest. But, it can be a good way to let people know what's going on and have a better chance that they see it.

Ask for feedback, ask a question, and solicit input on program development: Again, this is another one to use only every once in a while but it can be really useful to ask your subscribers what they want. You can find out more about what services they want, find out what other products and services they use (could be great for building relationships between your brand and others) and can basically ask, "How am I doing?" Sometimes, it can be scary to ask for feedback from your client base; it's nice to just revel in the nice things that people offer. But if you really want to grow as a business, it's critical you ask every once in a while.

In this section, we'll talk about the social media tools and suggested use for some of the major players: Facebook, Twitter, Instagram, You Tube and LinkedIn.

Facebook

Facebook has become a staple for the yoga community as a way to meet others, connect with students, stay up to date on classes and events, learn about the practice and build a community. Along with all of these things, it's also been a great way to build a brand, especially for the independent yoga teacher. Facebook gives everyone an opportunity to share their schedule, their teaching style and a little (or a lot) about them as a way to distinguish themselves from the crowd. It has given any teacher a platform to share thoughts, inspirations, pictures, videos, articles, blog posts- you name it. When used wisely and with a strategy, it can be a wonderful tool to help you build your business.

Facebook has two ways to build a profile: one, as a personal profile, which is the more common use for Facebook. This is the typical use for people when they sign up. But there are, of course, other options, like building a business page. Facebook gives you several different options for kinds of business pages. The categories are: local business or place; company, organization or institution; brand or product; artist, band or public figure; entertainment; cause or community. As a yoga teacher, you can certainly use your personal page as your business page and essentially build knowledge about your teaching and related activity off of that page. Another approach is to build a separate business page and use this as a way to build awareness. Even if you don't think you have a "brand" per se, know that YOU are the brand, like it or not, and when you're in the public eye, everything you do will be assumed to be part of the brand. For this reason, it may make sense for you to separate your two pages, if not for the mere reason that you might not want people who are not personally associated with you to see pictures of your latest birthday party or posts that are related to your personal life.

One caveat to add in here: assume that everything you post will be seen by everyone and anyone, even private messages, or those that are messages sent via any of these social media sites. We must operate with a mindset that assumes that anything we post could be viewed by anyone and would not raise concern. This is a great rule of thumb for anyone, and certainly when we think about the damage words, pictures and posts can have, we recognize we don't want anything we post to potentially be of harm to others or ourselves.

Having said that, and in going back to the original discussion, whether or not you decide to build a separate business page or not, there are general things you can do through Facebook:

- Let people know where you're teaching
- Tell them about special events you're hosting
- Post informative pictures and videos providing pose instruction
- Post articles and blog posts you've written
- Post other's articles and blog posts as they relate to your business mission
- Support others in their endeavor to create awareness around their brand
- Support others' teaching
- Share personal thoughts that may be inspirational or helpful to others

- Post pictures of events you're attending

There's obviously a great deal you can do on Facebook but one thing to keep in mind, especially if you have a business page: have a point to what you post. Try to always add value by posting something with your customer in mind. Yes, it's wonderful to share and this is a huge differentiator for any of us that are on line trying to build awareness of our brand. But, if your Facebook page is all about you and not about your customer, it doesn't add value to their day (Note: this is different from your personal page, where you can post what you'd like, although if you're also in business for yourself, be careful about what you post).

Twitter

Twitter is a microblogging tool that gives you 140 characters to share your thoughts. It's a fast read, obviously, and one that requires that you be savvy about what you want to share. Just as with Facebook, it's helpful to focus on providing value to the reader versus sharing just about yourself, giving unsolicited advice, promoting yourself non-stop or of course, trashing others. Use it more as an informational tool; for yoga teachers, we can use it to inform people on a daily basis about our schedule for the day, share articles we've written or articles others have written that we like. You can basically do everything you do on Facebook but you need to be much more judicious about how much you write.

One note: sometimes people wonder if they should have a Twitter profile if they have a Facebook business page. My thought is that it's helpful to be on as many of these social media sites as possible but you must have all these sites link off of your own website. Your website should be the hub for your business and anyone visiting your site should be able to get to your social media pages from your site.

Instagram

I really like this tool because it's basically all pictures. For a yoga teacher, that gives you a great visual platform to share your message and express yourself. The challenge, now that we're onto the 3rd social media tool is that if you're on all three, you'll basically have duplicate posts on all three sites if you choose to post the same content on all three. This isn't necessarily a bad idea, as you may have different followers on each site. But for those followers that track you on each site, they're going to see the same thing from site to site. This is even more of a reason to use a bit of discretion when posting in terms of just the sheer volume of your posts.

The other neat feature to Instagram is that you can post 15 second videos. Now, while this isn't necessarily groundbreaking, it's very cool for your subscribers to see live content every now and then. For yoga teachers, this gives us a way to post a transition to a pose or teaching we're doing, maybe in a cool location (make sure if you are taking video of children or adults in practice, you get their agreement to be in your post).

YouTube

Since we've talked about Instagram's video feature, let's talk about the cornerstone of free video content on the internet: YouTube. YouTube provides you with up to 15 minutes of time to post free video content. This is wonderful for yoga teachers because you can post informational videos, practice videos, videos with other teachers and training content as well and you have more space and time for your content to be expressed.

For these videos, I use a Flip Camera and have a standard set up for the camera in my living room. I always use the same camera angle for all my videos so they have a consistent look and feel from video to video. This allows each video to have a homegrown look, which is important so they look approachable (versus sterile) but the look of all the videos as you view the table of contents on YouTube looks professional versus scattered since they are all recorded in the same place.

It's important that you build a video page on your website. While your video content will be hosted by YouTube, you can embed the link for each video on your own website. This is critical in terms of building your business and the connection of your clients to your brand. If your subscribers/followers only see your videos on YouTube, they may be distracted by other links presented on the page where they're viewing your video. When you post the link direct on your own website, if visitors to your site watch a video, that is all they will see. This is yet another reason to build your own website and have all your social media pages and content there as well.

YouTube collects and tracks subscribers for you just like Facebook, Twitter and Instagram. When you post a new video, each subscriber will get an email alerting them that you've posted new content. You can also include a personal message with the video so your subscribers get the video and an accompanying message.

One special note: Insert a link in all of your videos to your own website. This way, when someone is watching your video, they can directly connect to your website and join your mailing list if they so choose.

LinkedIn

LinkedIn is the business profile and networking site that will allow you to create and maintain a professional profile. This is important for not only your professional career but also your yoga professional career, as it gives you a web page dedicated to your education and career off of which you can build a network.

As yoga teachers, we may come to yoga teaching during or after a business career that includes many different things. These should also be included on your profile, along with your teaching jobs.

LinkedIn also tracks connections you have and allows you to connect to others. You'll get unsolicited invitations to connect to people and you can use their search feature to find people you know or find people that work for certain companies, studios or other locations.

Other ways to build brand awareness:

- Writing articles for online publications on yoga or general health and wellness
- Share content from other people's sites, if they share a similar goal or clientele as you (note: this must be done authentically)
- Suggest friends like your page by sending invites via Facebook
- Intelligently contribute to online conversations or comment on related articles
- Tell your students about your social media pages (discreetly) when

you post articles that might be of interest
- Be consistent! Use similar content, brand messages and information across all your social media sites, again, all stemming from your website as your "business central"

Things to re-consider before doing:

- Asking people to "like" your page (note: this is different than using the invitation function mentioned above)
- Asking people to help you get to a certain number of fans
- Sending people unsolicited requests to sponsor you, join your fan page, link to their page
- Asking students to join your social media pages after class (in other words, outright asking versus adding value, i.e. offering an article that is posted for viewing)

Closing Summary

Remember that despite all of these new tools, nothing beats the impact of quality face-to-face interaction and the power of word-of-mouth marketing to help you build your brand. Keep that at the heart of all that you do and use these electronic tools to meet new people and reinforce your value.

Chapter 9

Essential Tips for Teaching

Focus

It's impossible to learn how to teach yoga only from a book. Learning how to teach yoga is part experiential, part academic, part heart and soul, and part practice (and lots of other things). But once you've built a solid practice and have completed your Teacher Training, it's helpful to be able to crystallize some of the highlights from teaching yoga into a short list.

The challenge when you start teaching is that you've got so much in your head from training, that it's hard to identify the important things that can help you when you step into the classroom. I always suggest to new teachers that they should start teaching as soon as they are done with training, otherwise fear can take over and paralyze you. Once that happens and the longer it goes on, the harder it is remember the elements of teaching that are necessary for expression.

Below, you will find some essential tips for yoga teaching. These tips are agnostic with respect to yoga style and cover a variety of areas: tips for keeping yoga safe, tips on sequencing; tips on building connection and thoughts on the qualities of a great yoga teacher. This is, of course, subjective and from my perspective, but will give you some idea of some of the characteristics you might aspire to develop.

Overall Considerations

Keeping Yoga Safe

There has been a great day of talk lately, debate really, about if yoga has created an increase in injuries related to practice. While I'm not going add to that conversation here, it's helpful for us as teachers to think about how we can keep our classes safe. The safety of our classes is in part, related to what we offer, but also must take into consideration the approach by the student to each pose. We can offer things in a particular way and make suggestions to individual students but ultimately it is up to them as to how they approach each pose.

Having said that, there are some general guidelines you can follow that can help keep your classes safe for everyone.

It's helpful to teach to who is in the room, not to the sequence in your head. In my teaching, I challenge myself to really "see" my students. As teachers, when we get more experienced, it's easy to lean on a sequence and wording for that sequence that allows you to go on autopilot. Maybe we're tired or not feeling well or we're not interested in teaching that day. Once we fall into this zone, we put our students at risk to a certain extent; they're here but where are we? What are we missing as we walk by, caught up in the sound of our own voice or the thoughts in our head?

We can also battle the voices we hear that have us wondering how we're doing, what they're thinking and these can act as a filter to prevent us from speaking from our hearts. It's great to have a 'go-to' sequence that frees you up to teach but if becomes a way to check out, it's time to re-evaluate things.

The less you say, the more they'll hear. People are pretty overwhelmed when they get to class. This could come from things going on in their personal life, career or it's just that they rushed to get there. Their ability to hear is hampered by the degree to which they can disconnect from all that's in their heads. The simpler you can keep the language, the greater potential your words will create the desired (safe) action.

Sometimes the greatest challenge is found in simplicity. I remember certain classes I've taken where the poses weren't the most challenging "technically" but the sequence was crisp, the teacher's words effective and in the stillness of class, you heard everyone breathing deeply. I found these experiences to be almost more challenging due to their simplicity. In these experiences, I was asked to focus on my breath, essential alignment and focus. The more essential you keep the practice, the risk of injury decreases to a certain degree.

Safe, effective hands-on assisting asks for your full attention to the student. As a teacher, we have the option to teach through words and to use our hands in the context of physically assisting students as a way to reinforce the primary action of the pose, deepen the pose or help a student who may be struggling with understanding the alignment. When we approach the student and in the actual assist, it's critical for safety that we focus on the student and his or her reaction to our touch. This can be challenging, as we also need to keep the class moving forward. A general rule of thumb: if you can't be there for the student, best to avoid assisting.

Only the truly present and connected student will know their edge. As students, we know (sometimes only in retrospect) when we're practicing from competition or a sense of pushing beyond our current limits. We know at that moment when we're not in our body; we're in our head. While we can't get inside the heads of our students as we teach yoga, we need to look for signs that students are pushing themselves into an unsafe position. Alignment is usually a helpful warning sign and many students, with an assist, will welcome the chance to settle into a position within a pose where they can feel their foundation better and breathe more deeply.

Tips on Sequencing

The sequencing you use will be a reflection of your training. There are many options from which to choose but there are some characteristics that are helpful to include regardless of the actual poses you offer.

A similar sequence from class to class gives you one less thing to worry about as a teacher, especially if you're new. As a new teacher, there's a lot to consider plus, there are all the things you've not thought of that will come up. For instance, there's the student who asks a question mid-class or the student who's injured and needs lot of help. These "unknowns" become so much easier to manage when you don't have to also think about what pose you'll present next.

Sticking to a regular sequence helps your students build strength and flexibility: Changing sequences often can make it harder for your students to build up their strength and flexibility. By staying with the same general movements, you help them get more solid in their feet, more proficient in the poses and start to stretch a bit more. This gets harder to do when you're changing the sequence from class to class.

A regular sequence helps your students become more efficient in their practice: "Efficiency" is an interesting word to use when describing a yoga practice but think about it this way: as a new student, you're unfamiliar with alignment. You're constantly moving your hands and feet in the pose to find the right position for your body. As you move, you're expending energy and this can tire a new student out faster than a more practiced yogi. As you become more adept in the practice, your hands and feet land in the right spot (for you) and you're able to move in a more efficient way. This preserves your energy so you can sustain yourself longer, without tiring. This becomes harder if the sequence changes from class to class.

Regular sequencing helps students (and you as teacher) connect to the meditative aspect of yoga: You've all heard the concept that yoga is a "moving meditation." As we bring students through the postures, we encourage them to slowly disconnect from their "thinking" mind and connect to the present moment. We also try to do the same thing as teachers so we can really see our students, give them the help that would be most meaningful in the moment and share from our hearts. This is harder to do for both parties if we're constantly thinking about what to offer next or what is coming next.

Regular sequencing gives you the space to be yourself, speak from the heart and inspire: Not every class is going to be one where you share a meaningful theme or story. In fact, for many classes, you may stick to the basics of alignment, breath and offering silence as a way to help students connect to their bodies. But regardless of if you teach a class from an "essential language" perspective or share more from the heart, it's aided by your commitment to sticking to a regular sequence. This will help you shine through more, will give your students a chance to experience you as a teacher and help them connect more to their own bodies.

Techniques for Building Connection

It's one thing to learn how to teach a pose, but it's another to express it in a way that facilitates connection between yourself and the students in class. This is, of course, the magical ingredient that can shift a class from being purely an exercise in alignment and can shift it to more of an expression of the heart.

As a teacher, we need to look for ways to build connection to our classes that are not just informational and instructional but also inspiring. This will take courage and fearlessness, as we work to open ourselves up to sharing and expressing from the heart. But it's so worth it as we see the signs of connection between our students and us and also feel it in our bodies. Here are some of the signs that you're building connection with your class.

You suggest an action and see it happen in the bodies of the students in class. One way to know you're connecting with your students is to look at their bodies when you are speaking to alignment and notice what happens. Do you see what you requested? Are their eyes wandering around? This can be a function of each individual and how present they are but it's also a function of what you're saying and whether it effectively cuts through the mental chatter to create the desired action (see my chapter on Using Essential Language for more tips on this). When you emphatically say, "Reach your arms high and take a big breath in!" and you see the whole class move in unison, you'll feel connected and so will they.

You have the courage to speak from the heart. There's a difference between teaching from the heart and teaching from alignment only. There are degrees of sharing that you can do as a teacher and there's always a balance you will be weighing between how much and what topics are too personal and what things are inspiring to share because they show vulnerability, compassion, empathy and warmth. When you have the courage (and this is what it takes for many of us, myself definitely included) to share from the heart, sometimes you'll see acknowledgement in the eyes of your students. You may also even elicit a response of some kind, a knowing chuckle or compassionate hum. But even without any auditory acknowledgement, just the fact that you took the leap is a step towards connection. Depending on what you shared, your students will know that you took a leap to share it and will feel a connection, even if the content was not necessarily relatable to them directly.

You are in the moment and have no agenda other than being present. Building connection starts with a commitment to being present.

This means that regardless of what's going on in your life in that moment, you make the choice to be present. This means you feel connected to your body, your breathing is steady and you are seeing clearly what's happening in the room. Your speaking voice is clear, your suggestions are relevant and your body language is one of accessibility.

Building connection to your class must start with being present. There's no way to build connection if you, as a teacher, are caught up in your head, problems you may be experiencing in the moment or if you are nervous about how you'll be seen or received as a teacher.

Being present as a skill starts as we sit in stillness and meditate. It continues on the mat during practice and these two practices give us the foundation that we then carry into our classes when we teach. This is why it's so important that as your teaching schedule grows, you continue to make time to practice. It's from your own personal practice that you can draw on sensation, a sense of stability and peace and this helps you as you teach.

You smile at the people in class. Do you ever notice how smiling can change your whole physical being? Unless it's a fake smile, smiling has a relaxing effect on the body. Think about it: you can tell if you're on the phone with someone and they're smiling. It changes the whole sound of your voice. Now, take that into the studio. If you smile, naturally, at your class and smile a few times while you're speaking, your voice will be lighter and you'll encourage your students to relax too.

The key is that is must be natural. If it's forced or fake, it comes across as insincere. As you're teaching, look for moments when you may catch the eye of someone and give them a slight smile. Or maybe you're telling a funny story and you naturally let yourself enjoy the humor in it. All these things will show your class that they don't have to be serious all the time when they're practicing yoga.

You refrain from judging and instead think: "how can I help?"
When you look at your yoga class, what's goes through your mind? Do you think, " Wow, look at these wonderful people doing something healthy? I'm so glad they're here," or do you think, "Wow, these people are all beginners. They're all over the place. This is going to be a hard class to teach!"

Of course, there are a number of variations in between. But the point is that sometimes our thoughts turn to judging how people look, their experience level, their clothes, their abilities or any number of things. These thoughts can affect how we come across to the class. For instance, if we're tired, lack patience and we notice a number of new students in that first Downward Facing Dog pose, we might sound annoyed or frustrated while teaching. If we can connect to positive feelings of appreciation and gratitude that we are being of assistance to others, it can completely change the way our voice sounds. The more we can communicate that we are approachable, non-judgmental and looking for ways to help, we build connection with the class.

For much of the class, our students won't even see our faces. They are upside down or turning right or left. It's for this reason that in order to build connection, our voice should communicate a willingness to help.

This "how can I help" attitude is best expressed by Deepak Chopra in his book, "The Seven Spiritual Laws of Success." The Law of Dharma, or purpose in life, suggests that once we combine the ability to express our unique talents with being of service, we will make full use of the power behind this Law.

You assist in class. One of the most obvious ways to communicate connection to your students is to physically assist them during class. While this may not always be possible, if you can fit it in, it's a great way to acknowledge them as well as teach in a different way.

While my chapter on "Essential Assisting Tips" will give you specifics around how to assist, in general, keep in mind that just as your voice must communicate a willingness to help, our hands must communicate this as well. In the exception where we're removing someone from a position that could be creating risk of injury, in most cases, we're assisting to communicate an interest in helping them experience the pose more fully.

You face the class and refrain from any practice, other than to occasionally demonstrate something. The question of whether or not to practice with your class is an interesting discussion to have with other teachers. Some teachers make practice a regular part of class, while others never practice at all. My personal preference and in my training with Baron Baptiste, I was encouraged to refrain from practice as much as possible. I have used this as a guideline over the years and it has never failed me. Refraining from practice allows you to see more, be of assistance more, get to your students quickly and build connection through really speaking to what you see.

Having said this, there are times when, in a class of beginners for instance, it makes sense to practice with them while talking them through the sequence. Especially in those first few Sun Salutations, it can be the difference for them between total confusion and connection.

As a general rule, if you hold back from practice, chances are you'll see more of what's happening in the room, this will allow your comments to be more relevant and personal. These things all help you to build a stronger connection.

You move around the room versus staying at the front. Depending on the size of your class, it may be hard to move around. Teaching bigger classes requires that we have oversight throughout the room so we're leading the group effectively. While it can be helpful to 'dive in' and assist students while teaching a large class, it can create a sense of disconnection because it blocks you from seeing the bigger picture.

Having said that, it is possible. I have watched some teachers build an amazing connection in a room of 100 people and they never left one spot. This comes from a tremendously deep well of experience and an ability to read people, read the group and make statements that hit home and break through the mental chatter to create action. In your general classes thought, if you can, move around. From a practical standpoint, this will help you get to students more quickly to assist. People will feel the energy you exude as you walk by and this can build connection as well. It also gives you a way to acknowledge each person's presence by assisting or passing them.

You talk to people before and after class and ask them questions about their practice and life. Getting to know your students even on a "name only" basis is a great way to build connection. This involves effort off the mat and outside the studio but it is a great way to help people feel acknowledged and appreciated. Asking that mom about her kids from class to class, or acknowledging someone for coming regularly will come back to you in spades through the act of people returning to your class.

The degree to which you chat with people is a reflection of your personality and comfort level with opening up to others. Hopefully, because you're teaching yoga, you have this to some degree. Remember that the best approach is one that feels right to you. Trying to be overly friendly, just like smiling too much in class, can come across as fake and insincere. Stick with what feels authentic and this will allow you to be consistent from class to class.

You are truly being yourself and no one else. They say that imitation is the greatest form of flattery. Ask any yoga teacher if they've ever sounded like the teacher with whom they've trained and they'll most likely say "yes" (if they're being honest). Especially when you're a new teacher, it's natural to sound like your mentor but over time, you'll build the confidence to sound more like yourself. Many years ago in my training, I remember we all sounded like we put on a "teacher voice" when we started to practice teach but in regular conversation, we sounded like ourselves.

Teaching in a way that's authentic to you, where you're truly natural and being yourself will feel effortless. It will feel grounding, relaxing and fun! How to do this is an art and comes with experience, mostly, but there are many new teachers who are able to immediately be natural, even in their newness.

When you can be yourself 100%, you will build connection to your class through the power of authenticity. There can be tremendous pressure students feel when coming to class, especially if they're new. If you're natural, open and authentic, the energy you exude will not only build connection but it will encourage people to do their best. They'll know through how you're speaking and what you share that you're speaking from both your heart and training and this takes courage. Through this approach, they'll not only feel a connection to you as a teacher but they'll feel an appreciation and be inspired as well.

Qualities of an Inspiring Yoga Teacher

While much of yoga teacher training is about the hands-on and technique, there are many qualities and skills that teachers build which speak more to their personality and who they are as a person. If we only teach from our training, our classes will be sterile and boring; if we're willing to show our true self, we will build connection with our students.

As you've taken class from a teacher you love or watched someone in training and noticed how effortless they made it seem, perhaps you noticed some of the qualities below. The idea of what makes a great yoga teacher is not a question that has right or wrong answer. The qualities important to you will be different for others. But there are some general things that from my experience and observation, I've noticed and feel are involved:

Courage: Great teachers are fearless. For those of us that have a fear of speaking in front of groups, being a yoga teacher puts us face-to-face with that fear but we do it anyway. Great teachers show themselves to others, express freely and take personal risks.

A need for approval/A fear of what others think: When you teach from a place of wanting the approval of your students, the whole student/teacher dynamic changes. This kind of need puts us less in the position of serving our students and more in the position of feeding our ego's needs and the needs of our ego have little to do with teaching yoga to someone else. Great teachers are able to proceed, acknowledge but resist the urge to let assumptions change their focus.

A sense of humor as well as humility: Smiling, bringing a sense of joy and love to your teaching, laughing at your obvious mistakes, sharing funny stories; these all keep the class light while maintaining the integrity of the process. Quality teachers aren't afraid to say, "I don't know" rather than make up an answer and are willing to show themselves with all their flaws in both the expression of their teaching as well in interactions with their students.

Creativity: One of the best times of each day in my initial training would be when I'd eat community meals and have the chance to talk to other teachers about what they're doing. Teaching in studios, opening new studios of their own, teaching in other countries, working for non-profits, teaching children, serving people that are facing many different kinds of physical and emotional challenges; the list is endless in terms of what my colleages were doing. Yoga teachers are creative in the form that their passion takes but they're also creative in the expression of the sequence, the way they manage their class, the way they may offer modifications and the inspiring thoughts they share.

A willingness to make mistakes: Teaching yoga can be messy. Arms and legs everywhere, sweat, personal expression, emotional release; these things aren't very neat. You're also leading a sequence, managing the room, and supporting beginners. In the context of this, you may make a mistake. A good teacher continues to move forward, learns from the mistake without personalizing it and looks for future opportunities to do it differently.

Passion for yoga and a strong desire to teach: It seems obvious but it's worth mentioning that simply loving yoga may not be enough. You need a passion for expressing both the poses as well as the coaching relationship that goes along with being a yoga teacher.

Passion for constant learning and ability to change: Teaching yoga is not static. How you teach in your first year will be different from how you teach in your second year, even around the same sequence. You'll change, what you emphasize will change but along with that comes a requirement that you're always looking for ways to increase both your academic knowledge of yoga as well as continue to push yourself to take personal risks in the areas of personal expression. This kind of personal expression only grows deeper and takes on a richer quality as you get more experience, as you learn from your mistakes, as you take risks, as you're willing to step into your full sense of yourself at all times, regardless of what role you're playing in your life.

Flexibility in mind: Having rigid thoughts about how we are, who we are, how others are and what is happening in the world is no way to live and is certainly cannot be the mindset of a yoga teacher. Yoga teachers work with people and people are dynamic, ever-changing beings. They need to be able to give and take feedback without making it personal, be able to think on their feet, be willing to take on new opportunities and be willing to let people make mistakes and show emotion, all without the need to control what is happening to meet their own needs.

Faith: Your own yoga practice is a beautiful expression of your faith. Every time you step on the mat, even during your deepest struggles, you affirm the resilience of the human spirit and the belief that things can be better. Yoga teaching, while a wonderful, inspiring and rewarding occupation can include different practical challenges as well as personal ones. But it is the faith on the mat that great yoga teachers show fully in their yoga teaching as well as in their lives.

Closing Summary

Your teaching will change over time but as you're starting out, keep the idea of being essential above all else. When you try to be fancy, complicated and popular, chances are good that things will fall flat, you'll get distracted and the energy of the whole experience will drop for you and the class. Instead, be clear in your language, essential in your word choice and present in your body and this will help you begin to develop your skills.

Chapter 10

Essential Assisting Tips

Focus

When we teach yoga, we use our voice and perhaps even our bodies in the pose to demonstrate what we wish to see in our students. In order to be effective, the description of the pose must be clear and our language essential (see the chapter on Using Essential Language). However, even with both of these actions, some students may have a hard time understanding the desired shape of the pose. Some people are visual learners, while others learn best from hearing instructions and yet others still learn best when someone helps them in the pose itself. This is where assisting can be a useful tool. Also, depending on the size and experience level of the class, assisting students may be a great way to build connection, deepen their experience and understanding of the poses and give you valuable experience working with students.

There are several critical aspects to assisting. They start with the aspect of assisting that touches on your objective for doing it at all and progress to various aspects of the practice. We'll review several different aspects of assisting here, starting with general principals and moving through the different aspects of assisting.

General Principles of Assisting

What is the primary action of the pose?

This refers to your purpose in touching a student in the first place. If you think about the main goal of assisting, it's to reinforce the action of the posture from the perspective of the student's experience. It might be to enhance or correct it on some level but it's always focused primarily on why they're doing the pose in the first place. The most basic reason to assist someone in a yoga pose is to reinforce the primary action of that posture.

What is the set up of the foundation?

Whatever is touching the mat is considered the foundation of the pose. This holds true regardless of the type of pose you're doing and whether it's on the feet or the head, for instance. We know that the steadier and sturdier the foundation, the greater the physical experience for the student and they are able to stretch and strengthen with greater ease. So, one of your main goals in assisting is to help them create a foundation that has greater stability.

What 3 instructional assists can be provided?

One of the main goals of assisting is to provide another avenue for teaching the pose. We've said what we want the students to do; we may also be showing them with our bodies as we do the pose with them. Assisting is another way to instruct the pose itself. If we do too many things at once it can be confusing. So, just as we don't want to overwhelm students with what we say, we don't want to overwhelm them with our touch. As you approach and observe the student, take the 3 most efficient actions you can to communicate instruction. This could be, in Warrior One, for instance, the following actions:

- Root the back heel down
- Center the hips
- Lengthen the arms

These 3 actions communicate what you might say to the student but do so with your hands.

What deepening assist can be provided, if any?

Although we want to be judicious in our use of assisting students in a way that takes them deeper into the pose, more out of a possible concern for injury, we can use these kinds of assists in a cautious way and create an enjoyable experience for the student. Having an assist that focuses on depth of the pose can be quite like a massage for a student and can allow for a deep release of tension.

Now that we've reviewed the 3 general principles of assisting, let's talk about some of the finer aspects of assisting. We'll tackle these by bundling them up into different sections that refer to the different aspects of assisting as a practice unto itself.

Physical Aspects of Assisting

Your goal is direction, not perfection

When you approach a student, rather than thinking, "Wow, look at all those things I need to correct!" Think instead, "How can I most efficiently help this student experience the main reason for doing this pose in the first place?" This again refers to one of the main goals of assisting I referred to above; that of reinforcing the primary action of the pose. Especially as a new teacher, we may get overwhelmed when we see a student struggling in a pose and may think just leaving them to figure it out is better than trying to help them correct the pose. Once we focus on the main reason they're doing the pose in the first place, it can help bring to mind 3 quick actions to reinforce that goal. For instance, a new student struggling in Downward Facing Dog might need these 3 quick actions to reinforce length in the spine:

- Bring feet closer to hands
- Bend knees
- Keeping knees bent, pull back on hips to lengthen spine

Also, once we tap into the idea that our goal is "direction, not perfection," it gives us a chance to soften our approach. We're trying to "direct" the student in the general direction of the posture, not force them into a shape that might injure them or just isn't within their body's range of motion to experience in the "picture perfect" way you may be imposing on them.

Make it meaningful or don't do it

Have you ever been in a yoga pose and the teacher comes up to you and does what I like to call a "drive-by assist?" This is the kind of touch that really has no purpose other than to touch you but without a purpose, doesn't communicate anything at all? This is one of the most damaging things we can do as teachers, not because we could injure someone but because it really just is an expression of us exercising what we might perceive as our ability to touch the student whenever we want. In fact, assisting a student by placing our hands on them is a huge privilege and one that should not be taken lightly. Even though our intent might not be to take advantage in any way, our lack of purpose communicates a lack of thoughtfulness. This can all be avoided by taking those few seconds, which is all you have really, to think of exactly what you want to do before you do it. While this can be harder in busy classes and for newer teachers, if you focus on one of the main reasons above for assisting in the first place, it changes the whole energy around your approaching and eventual touching of the student.

The bottom line, really, is just to be mindful about what you're doing. As soon as you commit to being mindful, this changes your energy also. It means that you're agreeing to be aware, you're focused on the person, your goal is to help not to harm and you've thought of a main focus for your touch. All of these things happen so quickly but they occur and with their occurrence, we begin to create what the Buddhists call "right action." You are taking the right action for the right reasons and with the right energy behind it.

Know your intent before you approach

This is related to the principle above about making your assists meaningful. It's important that you know exactly what your intent is before you approach the student. If you don't know, your physical presence and touch will communicate ambivalence and inexperience. This will also result in that "drive-by" feeling I referred to above. Having an intent means that you know exactly what your purpose is in touching the student to the degree that if they asked you in that exact moment, "What are you going to do?" you could answer it on the spot. If you'd stumble in that moment, then you know you're not ready and you should pass that student by.

It's much better to avoid providing half-baked assists rather than doing some kind of drive-by touching that only confuses and potentially makes the student feel uncomfortable. You should know exactly what you plan to do before your hands ever touch their body.

Start at the foundation and work your way up

Would you ever start building a house from the roof? The answer of course, is no. You'd start at the ground floor, in fact, even below that, with the foundation. Helping someone in a pose is based on the same idea, especially if your observation of the student is that they're fairly unsteady. Start with whatever body parts are on the mat and help the student become steadier before you suggest other actions that are further "up" the body, closer to the head.

Also, remember that if you want to provide a meaningful assist for a student who is really struggling, it's important to get them steady in their foundation first, even if it means you take them out of the pose and have them re-build it from the ground up. This works better in a private session when you have more time with the person but in a group class, especially towards the end of practice or at a time where you're having students hold the poses a bit longer, you will have those few extra seconds to suggest they step back into a basic pose, like Downward Dog for instance, and re-enter the pose from there. Done without reaction, minimal talking and some demonstration alongside them, this can be more effective than trying to help them adjust from the position they're in when you approach them.

Be steady in your foundation before you assist the student

Just as in an Airplane you hear the instruction to "place your oxygen mask on first before assisting your child," you need to be steady in your body before you provide an assist to someone. This means you need to be aware of your clothing and avoid tripping on your yoga pants as you move deeper into the assist (no wide legged yoga pants, please), need to be sure you're not going to slip on their mat or the floor, need to be practicing good body mechanics not only to preserve your body but also to have greater stability in your body while assisting the student.

This takes a split second and involves much of what we have already reviewed; you know what you are going to do, you know your intent, so you step up, get steady and provide the assist. Being in your foundation is in part, the key to being in your physical foundation but another piece is to know your intent. As we discussed, your intent is your purpose and once you have acknowledged that, you will be steadier in your physical body as well.

Decide what your focus is for the assisting: instructional, deepening, directive

I shared at the beginning of this discussion the idea of deepening assists and instructional assists. Along with those, there are assists whose purpose is one of direction; guiding the student into the direction you wish them to go. So, along with knowing your intent for the assist, you should know the general theme for the assist- to instruct on the pose's mechanics, to deepen the experience for the student by providing a bit more intensity in the stretch or providing direction towards alignment that will generate more integrity in the pose.

Let me take a moment to stop here and say that it may seem as if there are a number of things that you need to think of before you ever assist a student. You're right! There are quite a few things that go into assisting and while the list may be long, the more you teach, the more "second nature" these steps become. In reality, keeping these guidelines in mind allows you to make sense out of situations that might seem overwhelming at times. Especially for new teachers with beginning yoga students, it can provide much needed structure so both can experience the practice of yoga and teaching in a more fulfilling way.

Your goal is to help, not to hurt

Of course, no one would ever intend to hurt a student. However, depending on how zealous you are about bringing the student into alignment, or perhaps in your zest for providing a deep assist, you might inadvertently create discomfort for the student.

Also, one of the big areas where this is possible is in the case in which you don't know much about the student in terms of their physical condition or there possibly is something going on in the student's body that is underneath the surface and can't be seen visually in terms of how they hold their body. If this is the case, you could create discomfort by providing a deep assist and triggering this uncomfortable sensation.

Also, for students that might be experiencing any mental challenges, such as depression or anxiety, assisting someone in a pose could bring on feelings of pain or discomfort on more of an energetic level as well as physical. This could be felt in the form of sweating, increased heart rate and feelings of panic. This also would pertain to someone who has a fear of being touched, due to something negative they have experienced.

There is also the situation where you move too quickly or perhaps you're unsure of your intent. When we're in a rush or aren't connected to what we're doing, all of these situations could possibly create injury to our students.

In all of these situations, the solution is to be present, to know your intent and to be conscious of your main goal: to help the student experience the practice. The other key aspect of assisting is to watch the student's reaction as you're assisting them. Again, this is all happening very quickly but if you are diligent and attentive, you can notice things like increased breath rate, stiffening up upon touch or a grunt or a groan that does not appear to be one associated with a feeling of acceptable stretch. In all of these situations, the first thing to do is to back off and allow the student's body to return to it's neutral state and remain nearby in the event they have questions.

Provide hands-on help that reinforces the primary action(s) of the pose

When in doubt, assist in a way that reinforces the primary action of the pose. This takes us back to one of the main reasons to do an assist; to reinforce the main focus of the pose. This is always a good thing to keep in mind because as a teacher, sometimes we can get distracted by other things happening in the room (or in our heads) and as we approach a student to assist, our minds can go blank or worse yet, we get anxious and nervous about what to do. In these moments, we need to go back to the basics; that is, why we're there in the first place. And when you apply this concept to assisting, the one thing we're left with is the primary action of the pose.

This can also be a useful technique when you're assisting a large group and you don't have time to do a lot of fine-tuning with the student. Think of a primary action assist and use it with all the students as they are in that one posture.

Keep in mind that reinforcing the primary action of the pose depends on having a steady foundation. In some cases, your assist might need to be more on the gentle side or you may need to suggest a move for the student into a steadier foundation before taking them a bit deeper into the pose.

Be creative

Working with people in the context of yoga requires a great deal of creativity. The poses each have their alignment but each person's expression of the pose, their ability to move their body into the general shape of the pose and their flexibility and strength will differ. Also, each person's ability to understand the alignment through the spoken word will differ as well. For all these reasons, it's important that as teachers, we keep an open mind to being creative so students of all levels, abilities and physical capabilities can experience the practice.

Being creative can mean many things. It might mean using props to help a student experience the pose; in fact, it might mean using more than one block or folding a blanket in a creative way to support the student. It may mean showing the student as well as explaining how to do the pose. It could mean creating a custom sequence that supports the student in terms of their abilities as well as what they wish to focus on from a yoga perspective. It might mean stopping the class to walk through a pose or particular part of the sequence so students can understand it. We use creativity a great deal when we teach yoga to children; the poses are the same but the way we present them might involve games, singing, using special props like balloons or bean bags. Most of all, regardless of the age of your students, being creative as a yoga teacher means being open to all students, all expressions and letting go of your idea of the "right" way of doing the pose. When we approach things with an open mind, we soften our edges (especially if we tend to be a perfectionist) and it allows us to be more focused on helping and less focused on correcting.

Have props at the ready

Nothing is worse for a teacher than needing a block and not having one nearby. Part of your role before you begin teaching is to set up the room in such a way as to facilitate the student's experience. This means you need to think ahead as to what you'll need. If blocks are kept in the back of the room, grab a few to have near you. If straps are out of the way, do the same. Keep your eye out for newer students and if they don't have a block, quietly place one by their mat during the first part of practice. If blankets will be used in the practice, make sure they're nearby as well.

Encourage modifications

Often, students will resist modifying a pose because they think it's an illustration of their lack of experience. The reality though, for many students, is that modifying the pose will allow them to go deeper because they'll have more stability and greater overall integrity in terms of muscular positioning. When assisting a student who is a bit unsteady or appears to be uncomfortable in the pose, suggest a modification. This might mean you whisper something to indicate what position you wish them to take (something like, "drop your knee") or it could mean you offer a prop, such as a block or a strap.

When you move a student into a modified yoga pose, it will help you from an assisting perspective because they'll be steadier in the pose. This will allow any physical assisting you provide to be more effective. Creating length in the spine, or twisting movements for instance, will have greater depth because the student will have more integrity and stability in their body.

Use breath to deepen postures as tolerated

One of the really neat aspects of assisting is the synchronicity that can be realized between student and teacher. This can be seen just through the normal course of working with a student in any pose but in certain twisting poses, we can use the breath to help the student experience a bit more depth. If you're watching the student's breathing rhythm, you can suggest without words, that they inhale to lengthen the spine and the exhale to twist the spine, using the obliques and other muscles around the spine to create a deeper twist. Your hands will reinforce the actions they are already taken so the coordinated effort between the 2 of you creates the synchronicity.

Show, don't speak (unless really necessary)

One of the key qualities of an assistant (whether you're assisting while teaching or just assisting) is that your movements should blend in with the practice. Your assists should not break the students concentration, should not be a distraction and should only be there to enhance their overall experience. Therefore, in order to communicate what you want to express, the primary way is to use your hands. As soon as you speak, you'll break the student's concentration and practice.

So, this is another place where creativity comes in handy. Use your hands to point to where you want their feet to be, for instance, or use your finger to gently nudge their hip or knee in a directional assist. Perhaps use your own body to show them what you want them to do (this also may be a bit distracting but done without words can be effective).

As a last resort, you may need to use words with a student to communicate the desired action. If done judiciously (as in, not a conversation) this can also be effective. You can even use words while in a group setting as long as you keep your voice low and phrasing short.

Things to consider for yourself

Be present

You would think this goes without saying but it's still helpful to note. Being present as a teacher means seeing what's in front of you and speaking to what you see versus some script in your head that you've rehearsed. Being present when you're assisting means to look carefully at the student both when you initially approach and as you are assisting. It can be dangerous as well as uncomfortable for the student if you're assisting in a vacuum. This means you approach and you have a particular assist in mind and you provide it, regardless of what's happening right in front of you.

This can happen when we are newer, when we are not present, when we're nervous or distracted. It can happen when we're assisting more out of a need to please or a need to create a sense of connection. As teachers, assisting can sometimes be used in any of these situations and more often than not, the student will feel your lack of attentiveness in the quality of your touch.

Take a moment to prepare before you place your hands on any student. Remember always that it is a privilege and it comes with great responsibility. You would be better off avoiding the assist rather than providing one when you're feeling distracted.

Stay neutral despite feedback to the contrary

Depending on your personality, one of the harder aspects of teaching is to stay neutral despite feedback from students that might upset you, make you feel angry or frustrated. We can also take things too personally when we teach when in fact whatever the student is doing has less to do with us and more to do with them. In fact, everything the student does while practicing has to do with them. This might seem obvious but when we assist a student and they have different reactions, it's easy as the teacher to have a reaction as well.

Take the case of the student that you believe needs to modify or use a block and upon your suggestion, they don't take that action. This might be because they didn't hear you. But, if you're right next to them and you give them a block and they decline, you might take it personally. You might have a reaction and feel that you're right and they're wrong. You might get angry that they haven't followed your suggestion and might start to make assumptions about the kind of person they are and why they might be so stubborn (if you've read Don Miguel Ruiz' book, "The Four Agreements", you'll recognize that much of this language comes from that book).

The bottom line is that regardless of what the student does, you must remain neutral and steady. The more you get involved in why the student is reacting the way they are, the less effective you will be as a teacher. Stay neutral, regardless of the feedback you get from the student. This will save you in the sense that your assumptions could be totally wrong. Unless you're working one on one with a student (and even then, you might not want to ask) it's impossible to understand, in the moment, why a student might react the way they are to your suggestion. Provide the suggestion and keep moving forward. This technique also ensures that you can continue to be there for the whole group. The more you get involved in what's happening with that one student, the less you can be effectively teaching the group.

Wash hands before and right after class

This sounds obvious but be sure you wash your hands both before and after class. Enough said.

Be clean and aware of any open cuts or scrapes on students

See what you're looking at when you're assisting a student. If there are cuts or scrapes on their body, avoid touching those places. This is for your protection and for their safety as well.

Take care of yourself by hydrating and resting appropriately

When I was a teacher in training, I had a few shifts each week of assisting a senior teacher. My role was to assist only while he taught class. While you might think this relieved me of a significant part of the process from the perspective of "energetic demand," think again. Focusing on assisting only can be very intense and energy depleting. Make sure when you're assisting (and teaching) you're well rested and hydrated. If you're assisting and not teaching, take a moment or two during class to have a drink of water (I used to set my water bottle in the room in an inconspicuous place so I could get to it while moving through the room).

Just as we need to be aware of over-working ourselves as students, we need to be aware of the same when teaching and assisting. If we're tired and depleted, we won't be of help to anyone, least of all ourselves.

Arrive early to set up and be available after class for questions

As a full time yoga teacher, chances are, you'll be rushing to and from classes. This might not provide the ideal situation for arriving early or staying after class but if you can, take the time to do it. Many studios will ask teachers to be onsite at least 30 minutes before class, whether or not you have an assistant. This time can be used to check the room, place props where you want them in the studio and be available for any initial questions students might have. Sometimes students will let you know of injuries they have before class and it's a perfect time to give them a few tips about how to practice with their injury.

From an assisting perspective, it gives you time to set up the room with the props you'll need, gives you time to set up your mat and make sure that the room is clean and clear of anything from the class before. It also gives you time to relax and get centered and prepared for your work ahead. This is always harder the more rushed you are so this lead time will give you a moment to relax and check in with how you're feeling.

Establish a pattern within room to allow for a flow among students

If you're assisting another teacher, it's important to have a flow or pattern you'll be using in the room so you can get to each student. I used to assist large group classes of 60 or more people and in this kind of situation, you're basically working from one corner of the room to the next and up and down the rows until you get to the other side. When you're assisting as well as teaching, it can be a bit less organized as you're not so much focused on getting to each person as much as you are focused on helping those that need your assistance.

However, if you are teaching and assisting as well, at least walk the entire room so you are able to at least see each student close up and establish more of an "energetic connection" between you. Ideally, you'd get to assist each student but sometimes, this is just not possible.

Wear the right clothing for you

Yoga clothes have changed a lot in recent years and it can be more and more challenging to find clothes that are appropriate for teaching and practice. From the perspective of "appropriate" it only means that you wear something in which you can easily move but what you're wearing won't easily move on your body.

Things to think about include pant legs that are very wide and might induce tripping, loose fitting yoga tops or any other piece of clothing hanging off the body. I've become pretty fond of yoga leggings instead of wide pant yoga pants and find that they not only allow me to move more easily through the room but are better for demonstrating postures.

Get CPR and First Aid Training

As an assistant and a yoga teacher, it's important you are familiar with basic first aid as well as cardiopulmonary resuscitation (CPR) in the event you need to assist someone who is injured in class. In many cases as a teacher, you may be the only studio employee onsite at the time of your class and therefore, you need to be familiar with at least the basic factors involved in assisting someone should they become hurt. In most cases, this might involve a strain or sprain or possibly light-headedness due to dehydration, which can occur in heated yoga classes.

About the teacher

Keep in eye contact with teacher

If you're assisting another teacher, your role is not only to help the students in class but it's also to be an extra set of hands for the teacher. This might mean working with the heat or the lights, giving a prop to a student when the teacher gives you a look to indicate a prop would be helpful or could mean managing music before, after or during class.

Also, being an assistant for another teacher means you must think ahead and anticipate the things that might arise that could create disruption for the teacher or the class. Examples include a student coming into class late, a new student coming in and wandering around, not knowing where to place their mat or a student who is ill or distracted causing distraction other students. Your role is to recognize that what is happening in that moment might lead to other actions or situations that need to be managed before they occur.

As you're assisting students, it's critical that you keep in eye contact with the teacher as well as watch what you're doing. This is really an art but great assistants are able to do both. You need to be there for the student but also keep in mind that at any point the teacher may need you to do something and he or she won't be able to stop teaching to say whatever it is. Over time, as you assist a teacher regularly, you will develop an unspoken language and you'll know just via a look what the teacher needs.

Working one on one with a teacher as an assistant is a wonderful way to learn. It's also a great way to be of service to the students and see how the practice of yoga is expressed in the body. If you have never worked with a teacher in this way, find out from your local studio if they have an assistant program and offer your services. Also, the best place to start is to assist the teacher that trained you in your basic 200 Hour Program.

Take shavasana by sitting at the back of the room, within eyesight of the teacher

One additional note about working with a teacher as an assistant: Make sure you keep within eyesight of the teacher even at the end. I was trained by my teachers and agree that being in the back of the room, sitting quietly, but eyes open, is best.

About the student

Know when to back off

Sometimes as a teacher, we can get so focused on having the student "do it right" that we can keep adjusting someone even after the adjustments are effective. Just as stringing too many phrases together verbally can overwhelm a student, too many adjustments do the same thing; they just overwhelm a student, confuse them and can actually create resistance. So, just as you would with your verbal instructions, watch how your physical adjustments land on your students. Watch their face for reactions, watch their breathing patterns as you adjust them and be aware of the bigger picture; meaning, don't get so caught up in the details of what you're doing to the point where you lose sight of the fact that you're working with a person and need to be aware of their reaction to what you're doing.

Also, keep the general guideline in mind that you're there to assist people in the pose they're in, gently guiding them into alignment and certainly out of something that is unsafe. Your role is not to bring them into any kind of "perfect pose." Your role is to help, not to harm. Even if your intention is to help, if you overdo it, it can come across as harmful.

For deepening assists, watch student reactions before proceeding

We discussed the kinds of assists earlier in this chapter. Keep in mind that having a general approach to assisting that is more focused on guidance and direction can be just as effective and even more so, than working to move someone deeper into the pose. Some teachers are known to focus more on taking students deeper and while this can be enjoyable for students and another way to express the pose, it comes with a deep responsibility to stay aware of what you're doing and the student's reaction. Just as you don't want continue assisting someone once it's lost it's effectiveness, you don't want to take someone deeper into a pose if it's going to create harm.

The challenge as a teacher is that you won't often know if you're creating a harmful situation. Some students, in their interest in pleasing the teacher, will mask signs of discomfort. Also, sometimes students will be experiencing discomfort at the origin of the muscle, perhaps near their sitting bones for instance in a forward fold, and as you push down on their back to deepen them into the fold, they may be experiencing some pain but you won't know. The best way to know is to watch their face for reaction but this gets harder if in the pose, their face is hidden.

Overall, the most conservative approach is to simply refrain from any deepening assists, except perhaps in Child's Pose. However, just one note: I once had a student that expressed feelings of anxiety while being assisted in Child's Pose, due to the compression on the back and the way it would push the face closer to the ground. So, with all assists, be gentle in your approach and stay open to feedback from students about their experience in the pose.

Encourage beginners to be in the middle or back of class; make them feel welcome!

As an assistant, it's your job to make everyone feel welcome and get settled. Especially if you are assisting a popular teacher where you know the room will fill up, you need to help get everyone set up in such a way that the open spots are clearly left open. This way, as students enter the room, they will immediately see where there are open spots and they can place their mats down quickly and with little fuss and distraction to other students.

Keep in mind that the general approach for students is to plop their mat down in the first available place, especially if they're new. First timers enter the room and may feel self-conscious and nervous and as such, just drop their mat so they can quickly sit down and blend in. So, look for those students that come in looking lost and help them to a spot. I even like to take their mat when they're checking in at the desk and set it up for them. You'd be surprised as how grateful they'll be to have you take care of that for them.

In terms of mat placement, it's helpful for new students to be somewhere in the middle or back of the room. Don't stick them in a corner; give them a center spot so they have people around them and in front to help them with perspective. If you don't have any spots in the middle or back of the room, ask a regular student if they would help and move to the front so you can give the new student their space. People will be happy to oblige so the experience is enjoyable for everyone.

Get beginners what they need for props; they will often not know

Along with helping them select a space, help a new student get the props they'll need. Select the right blocks and include blanket and strap as well. Help them place the props in the right spot around the mat, with the blocks at the front of the mat where they can quickly get to them during practice.

Environmental

Establish a clean environment for students

Along with helping students set up, it's important that when they arrive, they have a clean space in which to practice. This also holds for teachers as well. When you arrive, set up the space with extra props near your mat or the front of the room. These will be helpful in a pinch in case you need to give one to a student. Also, make sure the room is clean from the prior class. If there are props strewn around the room or the prop area in the room is messy, take a few minutes and clean it up.

Make sure there are tissues, paper towels or whatever is used to clean up after practice.

While you might think this is bit obsessive, it's part of your role to ensure students have an uncluttered space in which to practice. Uncluttered spaces will help them relax and focus more on their practice. Imagine practicing at home and being distracted by the dust on the table and dust bunnies under the couch! It's the same with the studio; it should be clean for students. Also, keeping the studio neat is another expression of your yoga practice; it shows care and attention to detail and mindfulness about the space.

Facilitate appropriate spacing between mats

One of the hardest things to do is get everyone set up in the room such that you have open spots readily available, as mentioned before. In some studios, there are mat markers on the floor and these show the students where to place their mats. Even if these markers are there, often students ignore them or aren't sure how to use them.

As students are setting up in the room, be in the room and show they where to place their mats. While this is less needed in the smaller studios that get a handful of students, it can be really helpful in the bigger studios that can fit upwards of 60-70 people per class and very helpful at popular class times, such as right after work or Saturday and Sunday mornings. One of the keys to suggesting mat placement is to stay neutral to students' reactions. Sometimes, people want to be in a certain place and have lots of props strewn around them, taking up more than one spot. Or, you may need to ask a student to move over a bit, while you get their mat in line with the marker and then you can fit another person next to them. The art of doing this requires you stay neutral and pleasant and move through the room efficiently and with minimal conversation.

Have extra towels available

This is critical for heated classes and even non-heated classes in rooms where blankets are not available. Towels can be used not only for sweat but can be used in lieu of a strap and can be used under the head or hip, rolled up, like a prop.

As you're setting up the room, get a few towels and have them in the front of the room by your extra props. In heated classes, they also come in handy around mats where there is so much sweat, walking around the mat has become unsanitary or slippery.

Also, sometimes students come to class with a brand new mat. It sounds like a good idea, but if it's really slippery, their first Downward Dog will bring to light that the quality of the mat they purchased was pretty substandard. Rather than watch them suffer, just pull an extra towel and use it under their hands. Or better yet, give them a rental mat.

Spiritual

You're neutral, but recognize that touch can trigger emotion

I will never forget the time I was assisted by a male teacher and broke out in tears. I was going through a difficult time, recovering from a break-up, and the touch of a man with his hand on my back brought up a great deal of emotion. He would not have known what triggered it and honestly, I was not prepared for it; it just happened.

As teachers, we have a great responsibility when we not only teach yoga but take it upon ourselves to touch a student. In many cases, we're not stopping to ask the student, "Is it okay if I touch you?" but are just assisting them in the class. Some students may or may not want this and if you're a teacher that only occasionally assists, your students won't be used to the fact that it's part of your teaching. You can ask students before each assist but that only breaks them out of their practice and starts them thinking about what's happening or going to happen. You can let people know before class starts that you will be assisting and if they don't want assistance in the pose, to just say, "no thanks," or give you a motion to proceed on to the next student. You can also encourage students to approach you on their own before class to let you know outside of the room that they don't like to be assisted. These days, there are even little wooden coins that are markers students place at the front of their mat. One side indicates they wish to be assisted and the other indicates they do not.

There is a great deal involved in the emotional side of assisting and one of the obvious areas we need to consider are those students for whom touch triggers traumatic memories. Students that are victims of abuse or trauma can experience a rush of emotion as you touch them and again, you won't know any of this is in their background unless they tell you or share with you that they wish to skip any assisting. In all cases, remain neutral to their feedback. This doesn't mean you say nothing or show no facial expression but simply means you refrain from taking it personally. Once we do that, we change our body language and our voice quality as well. Students will pick up on it and then you're both caught up in an uncomfortable situation that will only distract the both of you during class.

As you move through the room, assisting students, if there are any reactions from students, stay neutral. I always remind myself that I will never know what's behind their reaction unless they share it with me, so it's best not to assume anything and turn it into a personal slight. Just keep moving on with the main purpose being you are there to help.

Take care of yourself before class

As teachers and assistants, it's important that we take care of ourselves as well. If we're not rested, don't feel well or are aggravated, that all comes through as we are assisting others and/or teaching. Make sure you've eaten, are hydrated, have taken care of going to the bathroom, are wearing clothes that are suitable for your role as assistant and/or teacher.

Taking care of yourself is critical so you can be there for your students without distraction. Also, make sure your hands are clean and you have brushed your teeth recently. It's also helpful to drink water before and during class, discreetly, to keep hydrated. Being hydrated also helps stave off bad breath.

Also, if your struggling with something on a personal level, make a concerted effort to put thoughts asisde about whatever it is and connect to the task at hand. I can say for myself, even in times of struggle, it's been a relief to teach because it's given my mind a break from the problem.

Closing Summary

The ability to assist students, either while teaching or as a stand-alone activity is a critical skill to develop. It shows attention to detail, recognition that not all students learn through verbal instruction alone and provide you with another way to build connection with people. It comes with a responsibility to be safe, promote safety and awareness and also requires that we develop a sixth sense that allows us to read into students' reactions and let them guide us into different directions. Your ability to assist well and effectively will help you develop your skills as a teacher around anatomy, alignment, breathing techniques and communicating with students.

Chapter 11

Using Essential Language in Yoga Teaching

Focus

Yoga teachers have many things at their disposal to communicate the poses and the elements of the practice. We have speaking, demonstrating and assisting, to name a few. When it comes to speaking, we have what we say and also the tone, pace and volume. In this chapter, you'll learn how to use language effectively, so you can communicate with your class clearly and help them experience the yoga poses fully.

Overall Considerations

As teachers, we can express the desired actions for a yoga pose from a variety of perspectives:

- How the pose feels in our own bodies
- How we've been taught
- The desired action we wish to see
- What we have found to be effective in the past

The words we use to describe each pose can range from simple to complex and can be based on sensation, anatomy or appearance of the body in the posture.

Often, people coming to your yoga classes are in a state of sensory overload. The constant stream of information we're exposed to through radio, television and Internet, and the challenges of our jobs and relationships can leave people exhausted and overstimulated. Your job is to figure out how to cut through the chatter in their heads to seal the connection between what they hear and what you want them to do.

So, for instance, when you say, "Bring your feet together," you want to see them step the inner edges of their feet together. Try it in class this week; make that request and then look at your students. Notice the variation among students. Some of it might be due to anatomy; for some people standing with the feet completely together is uncomfortable. But for some, it's because they aren't listening. They may be looking around. They might be concerned about what's going to come next. They're self-conscious. They're worried they won't be able to keep up. They're thinking they have to push themselves to get the most benefit out of the class.

Once you realize this, you see that the words you use (and how you say them) are a prime opportunity to cut through the noise and help them take action. Some words are more effective than others in doing this while others work better at creating a sense of relaxation in the practice. Adjusting the tone, volume and pace of what you say can effect how it lands with your class as well.

The other factor that directly speaks to the idea of sensory overload is the need to speak clearly and succinctly. You can say, "Bring the inner edges of your feet together, feel the edges pressing and make sure they're completely together," or you can stay, "Bring your feet together." As teachers, we often make a request and then repeat it in a variety of ways, either because we feel the need to keep speaking or we hope that in one version or another, it'll hit the students correctly. But this conversational style can mimic what people are already getting in the rest of their lives; that constant stream of information where nothing really sticks and it's just background noise. Instead, try saying it once and look at your class. If the majority hasn't taken the desired action, say it again. After that, move on.

Let's take a closer look at the elements of communicating through our voice while teaching. The components include:

- What we say and how much
- The tone of our voice
- The volume we use
- The pace at which we speak

Let's look at each one of these areas separately.

What we Say and How much

There are many ways to say the same thing but each will have a different level of effectiveness. Each will impact the individuals in our class differently, so we need to work over time to remember the phrases that work better than others. The more experience you build, you will start to develop a repertoire of phrases that you know work well. Some will work really well with beginners and some will work better with more experienced students. However, the general idea is to find ways to communicate the poses that work well for anyone.

Keeping your words short can also preserve your energy. The more we say, the more energy we're using to say it. As a teacher, we want to sustain our energy throughout the class and leave feeling just as energized and relaxed as the students. One way to do this is to speak less and see more of how your words affect the class. The other wonderful impact this will have is that you'll give the students more space in class for silence. Silence in between phrases will give your words a chance to sink in. It will also allow your students to experience a sense of calm in class. Can you imagine being in a class where the teacher talked non-stop? You'd most likely leave feeling frazzled and anxious.

Check out these examples below. Speak them out loud as if you were teaching a class:

" Can you bring your right foot forward and point it straight ahead and press it down?"

Versus:

"Step your right foot forward."

Another example:

" Please reach your arms up really high so you stretch your spine."

Versus:

"Reach up and stretch!"

You can see in the second expression of each of these movements, it takes less energy to say the entire phrase and you can add things like tone and volume to emphasize the action.

Here are some effective, short phrases you can use to communicate different actions:

Press, as in "press your palms"
Squeeze, as in "squeeze your right thigh"
Push, as in "push your thighs back"
Reach, as in "reach up"
Stretch, as in "stretch your legs forward"
Lengthen, as in "lengthen your spine"
Lift, as in "lift your leg"
Open, as in "open your chest"
Feel, as in "feel your body stretch"
Spread, as in spread the skin on your palms

In our desire to be expressive, we may sometimes use words or phrases that are harder for people to understand. This can be because we're speaking from our own experience and the sensations we feel in our bodies. While these phrases and words may be spot on, they may be harder for people to understand:

Rinse, as in "rinse your spine"
Tilt, as in "tilt your tailbone forward"
Tip, as in "tip forward"
Wrap, as in "wrap your elbows in"
Spiral, as in "spiral up through the crown of your head"

All yoga classes are designed to bring a heightened sense of awareness to the body so we can start to connect moving in a particular way to feeling a particular way. This is how yoga can help us off the mat as well. Once we realize that softening the shoulders in a pose like Warrior Two brings a greater sense of ease to the whole body, we become more aware of how relaxing the shoulders during the day brings this sense of ease as well.

This heightened sense of awareness is one aspect of mindfulness. If we can pepper our yoga instruction with both action-oriented phrases as well as those that bring a sense of mindfulness as well, our students will leave feeling balanced and will build skills that will improve their health and decrease their stress throughout their day.

Words/Phrases to help relax and bring a sense of mindfulness to yoga:

Soften, as in "soften your shoulders"
Let go, as in "let go of your neck"
Drop, as in "drop your head"
Release, as in "release the tension in your body"
Gaze, as in "gaze softly"
Open, as in "Open your heart"

Tone of Voice and Volume

When I hear the phrase, "tone of voice", I think of a mother saying to a teenager, "Don't speak to me in that tone of voice." Teenagers often experience a range of emotions and the tone they use can communicate frustration, anger or impatience. All these qualities can be communicated through not only what they say, but also their tone of voice.

In my work with children, especially toddlers and pre-schoolers, I have found that using a soft tone is a great way to get their attention; in fact, it's much better than yelling. If you want a group of unruly toddlers in a yoga class to focus, try whispering a request to crouch down like a cat or a mouse. They'll fall right in line.

Through these two examples, you can see how the tone and volume can make a big difference with children of all ages. It works similarly with adults. While kids have a hard time focusing because they're highly distractible, adults can be also. So the tone we use can help us create focus, emphasis and can bring a grounding quality to our voice. A deeper tone of voice comes more from the gut, while a whisper is more in the back of the throat and has an airy quality. If you start to think about some of what we've already discussed around phrasing (what you say), you can begin to see how the tone you use can be paired with what you're saying. When communicating actions, using a deeper tone of voice can be effective. When communicating the more mindful qualities of practice, using a softer tone can pair well and grab their attention.

Try it now. Using a soft tone of voice, say the following phrases:

"Relax your shoulders down and take three soothing breaths."

"Soften the muscles in your neck and relax through the face and jaw."

Now, using a deeper tone of voice, coming more from your center, say these phrases out loud:

"Push down into the block with your right hand, take your left arm up high and twist!"

"Bring your feet together, drop your hips low and reach high!"

By speaking these out loud, you can see how tone and volume can bring emphasis. It wouldn't be appropriate to yell something like, "Take three deep breaths and relax in the pose!" That would be a mismatch and quite assaultive to the nervous system. Using a tone that can help you communicate effectively can increase the potential for you to see the action you've requested.

One of the things that tone can also communicate is how you're feeling. While that might be a good thing if you're in a great mood and loving what you're doing, it's not a good thing if you're frustrated or not feeling well. As a teacher, we have to watch how our tone can express our underlying emotional state. Part of being present as a teacher is hearing how you sound. A helpful tool to use to illuminate this is to record yourself while teaching class and listen back. You will be amazed at the kinds of things that come up as you listen.

Another aspect of volume to consider is the volume needed in order to ensure that everyone in the room can hear you. There is nothing more frustrating to a student in class than to be in the back of the room, by the heater or humidifier and all you can hear is mumbling somewhere from the front of the room. As a teacher, you need to ensure that you can be heard. If you're not sure, ask. Do a sound check at the beginning, asking, "Can you hear me in the back of the room?" This is always helpful in large classes. The other piece that will help is your position in the room. Front and center is usually the best place to stand when you want to be sure that you project well.

Pace of Speech

A good yoga class has the quality of a symphony. The poses are like the notes and each pose expresses a different aspect of the practice. There is a natural build up to a crescendo and then a slow decline down to the end of the song. Solid sequences are necessary to ensure that we build poses with a strong foundation and give people a chance to stretch the whole body before we start taking them deeper into twists and backbends.

As we embark upon this yoga journey with our class, we want the pace of our speaking voice to fit nicely with the segment of the practice on which we're focusing. So, for opening Sun Salutations, your pace should be energetic; as you move into the heart of the practice, your pace should be even and steady. Moving into backbends, your pace should remain steady but the tone should communicate energy and strength, while towards the end of practice and the hip openers, your pace will naturally slow.

As you teach classes of different styles, you will find that your pace will change to match the style. A restorative class has a slower, more deliberate pace throughout and a beginners class may start with a slower pace, as you take students through the basics and then pick up once you've built a foundation with them.

One Final Tip about the Voice

Remember as a teacher, you need to warm up the voice, just as an actor or singer might before a performance. If you're teaching in the middle of the day or evening, that might not be a problem as you've been talking all day. But when you're teaching first thing in the morning, chances are, you haven't used your voice all that much yet. Singing is a great way to warm up your voice, regardless of time of day. Pick a song you know and love and start slow. Sing by projecting from your center. Do this for a few verses until your voice sounds clear.

Closing Summary

Your voice is one of the key tools you have to communicate what you want people to do, build connection with the class and show yourself. Even though what you may be saying is instructional in nature, your personality and warmth will shine through if you're committed to being authentic. Use your voice as a tool to effectively communicate the wonders of the practice.

Chapter 12

Bringing Anatomy into Your Teaching

Focus

As yoga teachers, we're teaching a movement practice. As part of our teaching, we're referring to body parts, movements, joints, muscles, bones and other anatomical information. As such, it can be helpful to have a basic understanding of anatomy. Your role is not to treat any of your students but when they approach with concerns about their bodies, the body's response to practice or aches and pains that have arisen, it is helpful to have a general understanding of what might be happening.

Learning anatomy is best done through a combination of studying and attending workshops and trainings that focus on this aspect of teaching. There are many wonderful books, resources and teachers that focus on anatomy or provide specialty trainings on the anatomy of yoga. Here, I will provide some of the basics in terms of practical ways to bring anatomy into your classes. Keep in mind, the best place to start is with the basics: the structure of the body in terms of bones, joints, muscles and the different movements the body can make. However, I will provide some of the application of that information below.

Overall Considerations

Why bring anatomy into class?

There are many reasons that it is beneficial for students and teachers alike to understand some of the basics of anatomy. While yoga is both a physical and spiritual practice, one's movement into the spiritual side of yoga can be facilitated when one is grounded into their body and their physical practice is solid. Having an understanding of the basics of anatomy can help with this.

Understanding basic anatomy can help us avoid reinforcing unhealthy patterns of movement and help to create new muscle memories that reinforce healthy alignment. When you consider that most people come to yoga a few times a week, that's barely enough time to undo unhealthy habits they may have in the other hours of the day. However, if teachers are able to communicate the key anatomical positions and information in such a way that it's translatable to daily living, we can help to increase the self-correcting ability of our students when they're off the mat.

Here are some of the key factors:

It helps you practice with greater safety and stability. Once we understand how the body moves, the shape and construction of the spine, the size, shape and construction of bones and joints and how the body's stability changes based on it's relationship to gravity, we can approach yoga practice with a better understanding about how to go into each pose and create a steadiness. It also helps us practice with a keen awareness towards being safe.

It informs you about the mechanics of healthy movement on and off the mat. When we understand what makes for comfort in a pose, we can start to translate those actions into the day-to-day movements. We can create healthier patterns of movement, self-correct when we've shifted into poor posture, and find natural ways to relieve tension in the body.

It gives you information to protect against incorrect (or missing) instruction. When you're more informed about the basics of anatomy, this allows you to move through your practice as an educated practitioner, without having to solely rely on the teacher leading the class. Also, in large classes where it can be challenging to help each student individually or provide ample instruction it can be helpful if the student understands how to apply basic information to their practice.

It allows you to build strength and flexibility with less risk of injury. There's risk inherent in all kinds of exercise and that risk will vary depending on the exercise itself, the condition of the practitioner and the knowledge of the teacher and student. The more one understands the basics about anatomy in the context of movement (think of just the anatomy involved in things like folding forward or holding Side Plank

Pose) the greater the opportunity to create strength and flexibility in a healthy way.

It gives you the ability to apply yoga to help manage the impact of a structural shift in your body or a unique characteristic, such as being double jointed or having scoliosis. As students are more educated about the basics of anatomy, they are able to go into any group class and create customizations that allow them to experience the practice in the best way for them.

It helps you understand the anatomical impact of some poses compared to others. The other factor to consider in a group practice is that poses are offered that might not work for everyone's body in the most general way. While students don't need to do every pose, the general tendency is to try what's offered even if one might not have the proper positioning to enter and stay in the pose safely. Also, without a general understanding of anatomy, it can be hard to discern between one pose and another when it comes to the shape of the pose and what might be involved from a positioning perspective. Some poses are generally harder than others and require things like greater stability, flexibility or strength, but in addition, some poses move the body in ways that can create stress on joints or the origin and insertion of muscles. Additionally, some of these characteristics can be inherent in even basic poses, such as the risk of overstretching the hamstrings in Downward Facing Dog. Once we give students general anatomical information, they are better able to understand why the knee in Pigeon is potentially at risk or the vertebral discs are compressed in different ways, depending on the way the spine is bending and our body's relationship to gravity.

It's empowering. When we understand the basics of anatomy as it relates to the body and our yoga practice, we feel more empowered as a practitioner. We can feel as if we're taking a greater responsibility towards our bodies and can make adjustments in a way that acknowledges our uniqueness as a practitioner.

Basic Anatomical Landmarks as it relates to Yoga

Now that we've established some of the reasons to inform and educate about the anatomy behind yoga practice, let's review some of the basic anatomical reference points that can be helpful to know and on which to cue your students. When we teach yoga, we use words and phrases to orient people to certain parts of the body. Knowledge of these points is essential to create healthy alignment and to allow students to customize each pose as they see fit. As students, we hear the words and phrases and try to interpret where they are on the body or what action we are being asked to take.

We know from watching the class that everyone can have a different understanding of these body parts and actions. People come to class with a lot on their mind so the more essential we can be as teachers in our words, the better. It can be helpful to know some basic references so you can set up the alignment correctly.

Feet hip width apart: It's interesting to watch the class when you request people to stand "with feet hip width apart." In many cases, it can be due to the student not hearing the instruction or just being less diligent about positioning the feet in this way. Use the reference point of the hip joint and imagine a straight line down to the ankle joint, traveling down the outer thigh. Stack the hip joint over the ankle joint (you can use your lateral malleolus, that ball-like structure that sticks out of your ankle joint as reference). Be sure your knees point directly forward or slightly move them to that position, noticing if the tendency is to have the knees falling in towards each other ("known as "knock kneed").

Stacking hips over heels: Now that we've discussed the alignment of bringing the feet to hip width, we can take this foundation and when we come into a forward fold, create healthy alignment in that position too. As you have your feet at hip width and fold forward, bend your knees if you need to in order to keep the hips in line with the heels. The other tip you'll potentially need to use is to lift your sitting bones up. Working these two actions together will allow you to stack your hips over your heels. This position stretches the hamstrings and allows the upper body to relax.

Knees in line with the hips: As we work the concept of "feet at hip width" up the legs, we come to a related physical orientation, that of "keeping the knees in line with the hips." If you stand with your feet at hip width and your knees at hip width, arms at your sides, palms forward, you'd be in "Anatomical Position," that "home base" of positions where the joints are aligned. When we start to take the knees outside hip width, as in poses that have us in a squat, for instance, we're typically externally rotating our hips or opening the inner thighs. But in poses like Bow or Wheel, when the knees widen beyond hip width, we're actually decreasing the width available in our lower back for the backbend we're trying to do. This can make these poses uncomfortable and actually a lot harder than if we stay at hip width as much as possible.

Stacking the knee over the heel: There is a good amount of "stacking of joints" that occurs in yoga and stacking the knee over the heel is a common reference in poses like Warrior 1 and 2. In this position the knee joint is most steady. As the pose goes deeper in it's expression, the front foot may need to move forward to keep the knee over the heel.

Drawing the shoulder blades together: This can be an important action in many poses to allow one to open the chest. When we use the muscles called the Rhomboids, we are drawing our shoulder blades closer together. The resulting affect is to open the chest or what may be referred to as "stretching across the collarbones." This can be a helpful action to take in poses like Wheel, Locust, Bow and Upward Dog. It's also helpful to be aware of this action as you are sitting at your desk and possibly hunching over your computer.

Shoulders back and down: The shoulder joint is a ball and socket joint (like the hip), and its most stable position is when the "ball" part of the upper arm bone, the humerus, fits nicely into the "cup" formed by the shoulder blade or scapula. That "fossa" of the scapula holds the humeral head with the best support from the nearby muscles, ligaments and tendons when you relax your shoulders "down the back." If you hunch your shoulders up by your ears and then drop them down in a relaxed position and slightly draw the shoulder blades together using your Rhomboids as referenced above, you'll create a steady shoulder. You can use this for support in poses like Side Plank, Crow, Upward Facing Dog and many inversions like Handstand, that depend on shoulder steadiness to create safety and stability.

Top edge of the pelvis: The two pelvic bones join together in the back at the sacrum and in the front at the pubis. The top edge of the two pelvic bones forms a "rim" and the shape of the pelvis is bowl-like.

The word "pelvis" is derived from the Latin word for "basin." Teachers sometimes refer to making the top edge of the pelvis level or to "lift the top edge of your pelvis." This orientation is helpful in poses like Warrior 1 and 2.

Sitting bones: known as the "ischial tuberosities," these two knob-like bumps are on the bottom edge of both of the pelvic bones. They hit the floor when we sit down right on top of them. They're what you'd be sitting on if you were on Boat Pose (Navasana). You can tip them forward as you sit on them or stand or you can tip them back. Sometimes teachers refer to "sitting on the front edge of the sitting bones" in a pose like a Seated Forward Fold (Paschimottanasana) or "dropping the sitting bones toward the heels" in a pose like Chair (Utkatasana).

Tailbone: Known as your "coccyx," this is the final section of the spine. It's concave when viewed from the side and depending on the orientation of the top edge of the pelvis, can be either reaching back or "tucked" under. When the tailbone is tipped backward, it's known as "hyperextension" (too much extension). This orientation of the tailbone is commonly seen in people where the hip flexors (such as the psoas) are shortened, thus drawing the pelvis into a forward tilt in a pose like Warrior 1. A helpful correction is to lift the front edge of the pelvis and drop the tailbone down.

Center your hips: Since we've talked about the pelvis being shaped like a bowl, with the top rim of the pelvis being an anatomical reference point, we can now talk about how to center the hips. If you put your hands on your hips, while standing with the feet hip width distance apart, you will feel the top edge of your pelvis. If you bring both of your index fingers to your belly button, you can start to trace your fingers along the top edge of the pelvis. The two highest points, called the ASIS's (Anterior Superior Iliac Spine) are commonly called "hip points." These reference points become the markers for centering the hips or bringing the hips more towards a centered position (remembering that this instruction is a guideline, not something to hear and than shove yourself into the shape). As you hear "center your hips" you will bring the two ASIS's more towards the front edge of your mat (in a standing pose like Warrior 1 for instance). Your hip points would face directly down in a pose like Pigeon. Keep in mind that in order to center your hips, the position of your feet is crucial in order to assist you into this shape.

Lift the front edge of the pelvis: As students work with tight hip flexors, their pelvis is tipped forward. A good way to think of this is that if a person wore a belt with a big belt buckle at the center of their waistline, the belt buckle would tip down while they are trying to come into a standing pose such as Warrior 1, for instance. In order to help them stretch their hip flexors, like the iliacus and the psoas muscle, they need to "lift the front edge" of their pelvis.

Relax your upper ribs: In several standing poses, like Warrior 1 and Crescent Lunge, students may thrust their chest forward, creating a "caved in" back or lordosis ("swayback"). To avoid this, which will tip the front edge of the pelvis down and prevent stretching the psoas, relax the upper ribs. Place your hands under your chest and soften right under the chest and draw it slightly inward. At the same time, draw your belly in slightly to activate your rectus abdominus, the long abdominal muscle that runs up the midline of your body. These two actions will level your pelvis and help stretch your psoas (on the straight leg) without hyperextending your tailbone.

Internally rotate your thigh bones: In backbends, including Bridge, Upward Bow and Bow, it's helpful to keep the thigh bones aligned, internally rotated and the feet parallel to each other. To internally rotate your thighs from standing, stand with your feet hip width distance apart and rotate your inner thighs back. In Bow Pose, your inner thighs would roll up towards the ceiling and in Upward Bow, they would roll down towards the floor. This positioning keeps the lower back broad, which is helpful for backbends.

Applying Anatomy to the Practice

The application of anatomy to the practice is really where things can start to blend together. Once we understand the basics and start applying them to different poses, sequences and challenges that students face, we can start to make the information come to life. Here are several different Teaching and Practice Tips that take the anatomical information and apply it to yoga. Where appropriate, sources have been noted.

Teaching/Practice Tip 1: Create healthy alignment in the back during forward folds and when coming up to standing

Teaching or performing "rolling up to standing" compresses the soft gel inside the discs anteriorly (at the front), creating a dynamic known as "anterior disc compression." The degree of compression increases more if the hamstrings are tight due to the inability to lift the sitting bones. The bend in the forward fold is coming more from the lumbar and thoracic spine, therefore, it's better to come up with a straighter spine. This action protects the disc and prevents compression, especially over time. Keeping the spine as elongated as possible is also helpful when folding forward in any position.

A helpful reference about this movement can found by checking this URL: http://sequencewiz.wordpress.com/2013/08/14/rolling-up-from-a-standing-forward-bend-can-damage-your-spine/

Teaching/Practice Tip 2: Protecting the natural curves of the Spine

These natural curves of the spine are meant to be there. Extreme flattening of the back to the floor, as in hugging knees to chest or doing aggressive abdominal work will flatten the curves, especially in the lumbar spine. Also, tightness in the hip flexors, like the psoas muscle, can create an overly exaggerated lordosis ("swayback") in the lumbar spine.

Teaching/Practice Tip 3: Creating healthy movements in the spine when practicing

The thoracic spine, or mid back, can demonstrate less mobility than the other parts of the spine, due to its job to protect the heart and lungs. Also, the ligamentous connections between the ribs, spine and the sternum are very stable and provide only for limited motion. Because of this, movement in the thoracic spine, while possible in all directions, occurs only in small magnitudes.   As a result of its inherent stability, it can be hard to get movement here when practicing yoga. By contrast, the cervical spine is much more mobile because the vertebra are smaller and rotate with much greater ease. Therefore, care needs to be employed to moderate neck movements so as to not create instability.

Teaching/Practice Tip 4: Practicing healthy joint movements during yoga practice

The less mobile the joint due to its structure, the greater risk to the joint in poses that request a wider range of motion. Also, when joints are taken outside of their normal range of motion, this can put them at risk along with when joints are "locked." Depending on a person's mobility and ability to sense when these potentially injurious things are occurring, the risk can be greater or less.

Teaching/Practice Tip 5: Stabilizing the Shoulder Joint during practice

The most steady and healthy position for the shoulder joint is "back and down." Think of this as the opposite of hunching forward and letting the shoulders move up around the ears. When standing in Anatomical Position with the palms facing forward, the arms are externally rotated and thus the shoulders are naturally positioned in this healthy way. Also, with the elbows slightly flexed, it facilitates this shoulder position as well. However, when we internally rotate the arms, the shoulders start to move out of this position and the head of the humerus begins to push forward into the muscles of the shoulder.

To avoid this, especially in poses like Downward Facing Dog, Plank and moving from High to Low Push Up, wrap your elbows in by your sides. This activiates the Serratus Anterior muscle, which draws the shoulder blades apart and down the back.

Teaching/Practice Tip 6: Working with tight hip flexors

First let's look at the primary muscles that flex the hip. One of the major hip flexors is the Psoas Major. It originates in the lower back, at Lumbar vertebra 1 through Lumbar vertebra 5, continues on in front of the pelvis and inserts on the lesser trochanter of the femur. (the top of the upper leg bone). Its action is to flex the hip. This can be further described as lifting the upper leg towards the body when the body is fixed or to pull the body towards the leg when the leg is fixed.

Due to prolonged sitting, running, cycling and other hip flexion movements that we hold for a long time (driving, for instance) they get tight and shortened. As they get tight, the pelvis tips forward and compresses the lower back. This "tips" the person forward and now, to lift the arms and stand upright, the student has to overarch his spine, called hyperextension (think of this movement like sticking your tailbone out).

To correct this, you would lift the front edge of your pelvis. Think of this movement as lifting your belly button up so it's directed forward. You can also draw your belly button in towards your spine and create as much length as possible up the middle of the body.

Please check the URL to see a wonderful explanation of this:
http://www.yogajournal.com/practice/588/

Teaching/Practice Tip 7: Moving from High to Low Push Up

For many people, this movement is challenging due to a number of things. First and foremost, it is often because there is little knowledge about how to take the movements while keeping the proper alignment and engaging the proper muscles. Sometimes it can be due to a lack of strength in the various muscles needed.

Improperly performing High to Low Push Up, while frustrating, can also create a shearing force on the muscles, tendons and ligaments that support the shoulder joint. This force can create shoulder instability or worse, injury.

Let's first look at what someone may be doing when moving from High to Low push up:

- Shoulders ride up to ears, crunching the skin on the sides of the neck, "dumping" into deltoids
- Elbows winging out
- Scapula winging off the back
- Rhomboids overworking, drawing scapula together
- Head dragging down, leading with chin
- Dropping shoulders lower than elbows
- No action in the transverse abdominals ("cinching in")

When someone lowers into Low Push Up using a muscle in the back called the Serratus Anterior, there is the appropriate action of stabilizing the shoulder blades flat on the back. There are a number of complementary actions that need to occur in order to create the appropriate movement:

- Hug elbows into sides
- As you lower, slightly externally rotate upper arm bones
- Shift forward before lowering to create the right angle in the arms, elbows over wrists
- Push into the floor as in Cat Pose as you lower
- Activate core ("cinch in")
- Only lower shoulders to elbow level

This information should be credited, as with the previous examples, to the author. See the URL here for more detail:
http://yoganonymous.com/yoga-tune-up-maura-barclay-chaturange-article-yoga-practice-tips/

Teaching/Practice Tip 8: Getting the most out of Upward Bow Pose by using the Gluteus Maximus to extend the hip

When working in poses like Bridge or Upward Bow, we need to leverage the natural ability of the Gluteus Maximus to extend the hip. This muscle is the big muscle in our hip and the roundness of our seat. However, as it also works to externally rotate the thigh, we need to counteract its ability to do that. When we externally rotate the thighs in a backbend, we compress the lower back, resulting in compression of the lower spine.

In order to do this, we need to keep the feet straight and parallel to each other as we come into a backbend. In fact, we need to try to rotate our inner thighs down towards the mat. The muscles involved in this are the Gluteus Medius and the adductor muscles, which are the muscles that draw the thighs closer together.

Closing Summary

The art of bringing anatomy into your classes is an important part of helping people become more aware of their bodies and to help them understand how the alignment works. Bringing anatomy into class need not be a complex thing; it can be a wonderful way to educate and reinforce one of the more concrete aspects of yoga practice.

Chapter 13

Managing Challenges in the Classroom

Focus

One of the challenges of teaching any subject, not just yoga, is the situation of managing challenges in the classroom. Although you think you might prefer a class without bumps in the road, it's through teaching a challenging student or handling an unexpected question or issue in the moment that one can grow as a teacher.

These kinds of discussions should be held after the basic foundation of yoga training has occurred. This ensures that the basics around the postures, alignment, sequencing and other key aspects of yoga teaching have been completed. It is only then that this knowledge can be applied to the idea of teaching through challenges that may present.

Overall Considerations

Every yoga class you ever teach will be different. Just as every yoga practice you do yourself will vary, so will your experiences as a teacher. Even if you were to teach the exact same one-hour sequence every day for a year, there will be variations. The people in class will obviously be different; your description of the poses will vary; the pace, the energy in the room… these are just some of the factors that will change.

It's for this reason that I always encourage new teachers to use a standard sequence when teaching. This provides a degree of consistency for the students so they can learn and build muscle memory. In addition, it provides a level of stability to you, as a teacher, so you can be ready to handle whatever may arise that is unexpected. One of the best preparations for something unexpected is to take time to think about some of the more common scenarios that may arise for which you need to be "on your toes." Just as in an emergency, the better prepared you are, the more you can stay focused to handle whatever comes up.

Here are some common situations you may encounter that could potentially throw you for a loop:

You have a class with a few beginners and more advanced practitioners.

In this situation, you may be tempted to teach to the advanced students out of a concern that they will get bored if you stick to the basics. This approach may work for them but will most certainly be less palatable for the newer students. This situation may not be obvious to you until you start teaching the class, so you need to be ready in your head with an approach that you can use so you can stay on track, not drop the ball, leaving people hanging, while you freak out in the front of the room.

This is something you may find happening more these days as well, as new students take advantage of Group On and other discount deals as a way to join a yoga studio for the first time. This blend of student ability levels can present a challenge and unnerve a teacher. The approach that I like to use in this situation is to speak to the basics of alignment and foundation. Hold poses longer. Challenge the students to set their gaze, or drishti, and stick with it. Focus on moving lightly, like a cat, stepping cleanly from pose to pose without dragging the feet. Suggest people practice ujjayi breathing and focus on their breath in each pose. This approach will support a new student, will slow the flow down so everyone can access each pose and will most likely challenge a more practiced student who may be used to flowing from pose to pose without thinking any longer about these basic variables.

One additional way to be on alert that this scenario will appear is to keep an ear out as people are signing in for class. If you are doing your own check-in, you'll know who the new students are from the check-in process. Ask them to set up in the middle or back of the room so they have a good vantage point to see you and the others. If you're not doing check-in, be on alert as your colleague does it so you can welcome the new person and show them where to set up in the room. A new student walking into the studio for the first time will instinctively put their mat down in the first available space as a way to decrease their nervousness and self-consciousness. This often will be in the front and you'll want them to be more mid-room to have a better experience.

A student comes up to you before class and asks you to "Make today's class really hard!"

This can happen as you develop a more familiar relationship with your students. You want them to feel like they're getting what they want, but you also have to take into account the bigger picture as you're a group facilitator, not just there to meet the needs of one person. You also know as a teacher that the role of yoga isn't to present just the poses more commonly thought of as challenging and in fact, it's through the more essential postures that we are faced with the challenge of staying present and with the breath. The presentation of challenging postures may be already in your plan, may be a theme you're regularly working on with your class or something that might spontaneously come up if you feel it's appropriate in the moment (a sense you'll develop as you teach more). If none of those factors are present, it's not necessary for you to meet the needs of one person despite their request.

In these situations, stay calm, friendly and non-reactive when responding to the person. Sometimes, as yoga teachers, we put on our "people-pleasing" hat and we try to be all things to all people. This is an impossible approach and will only lead you down a path of frustration. You might say something like, "I love your willingness to take on a challenge!" Know that the spirit of this person is that they want to work hard. Challenge them through deep breathing, focusing, holding a pose longer and staying relaxed in each posture. These essential tools are critical for students to learn and often are overlooked as they strive to get into a challenging pose.

You're teaching outside a traditional studio and the client asks you to refrain from using Sanskrit or chanting before and after class.

One of the wonderful things about yoga's reach is that it has made its way into schools, businesses, private clubs and other settings outside of a yoga studio, where yoga is traditionally practiced. As a result, more and more people are learning yoga and more teachers have opportunities to bring yoga to these non-traditional settings and privately contract for the business.

When yoga is practiced outside a studio, the host or sponsor of the class may or may not be familiar with the practice and its key components. They may be looking at it as an exercise program and have little interest in bringing into the classes any aspect of yoga's philosophy, principles, language or sound (through breathing or chanting). As a result, you may feel insulted or angry, or perhaps may not have asked about this prior to starting the class. You may find out afterwards that your approach and actions are inconsistent with the vibe and flavor the client wishes to extend to the practitioners attending (this could also come up in regards to teaching children's classes).

One of the best things to do is ask about this before you start teaching for this client. Part of all my initial conversations with individually contracted clients like those mentioned above includes a discussion about the general tone and focus of the classes. Some businesses, for instance, want to use in-house yoga classes as a way to introduce yoga to those who have never tried it before. They may want the focus to be on the basics of breath and movement and less on the philosophy. It's important that you educate them on the basics that are non-negotiable: breath, focus and foundation. However, beyond that, you may be willing to hold off on chanting "OM" before and after class and may be willing to stick to English versus Sanskrit.

I usually share with clients that I like to finish class with the word "Namaste." I tell them what it means using the translation, "The spirit in me bows to the spirit in you." I share that this sentiment is more of an acknowledgement and a way to thank each other for practicing together. Using that description, most people usually agree that this is fine.

If you neglected to bring it up, and receive feedback after your class, try to stay non-reactive and calm. It's easy to get defensive and try to justify your actions and approach. Remember, your goal isn't to be "right" and make the client "wrong;" your goal is to try to reach a place of understanding and where you can continue to teach the classes in a style where you don't feel compromised and the client doesn't feel uncomfortable.

If, after discussion, you feel it's impossible to find a middle ground where you are able to teach freely, then perhaps the client isn't the right fit for you and your teaching. This would be rare, hopefully, but could happen. In that case, share with the client that you can help them find another teacher. Honor any remaining classes you have in the contract unless they are willing to let you walk away on the spot. Always keep the contact professional because you never know where this person will appear again in your life.

Someone asks a question out loud during class.

Everyone has a different sense of how to handle themselves in a yoga class. Some people automatically drop their voice down to a whisper from the minute they check in to the time they leave. Others talk loudly, bang around as they set up their mat and props and march around in the middle of class to go to the restroom or get water. For you as the teacher, this can be a real distraction as well as one to the others in class. Most students, when they have a question about a pose won't ask but will try their best to figure it out by watching others. This requires you stay alert and watch for alignment issues that need to be corrected in the moment. Even if you feel the message is only for a few students, it's always a good reminder for everyone.

Every once in a while, you will have a person who blurts out a question. It will most likely throw you off a bit, as you'll be in the middle of teaching and the question could jolt you out of your meditative state. My initial instincts as a new teacher were that I kept teaching and slowly moved over to the person to quietly fit in an answer just to them. But after a while, I realized this was unnecessary. Chances are, the question that person has is the same question that many others have. Also, in a way, it's wonderful to have someone ask out loud because as teachers, we're pretty much left to presume what our students are thinking through their body language and actions.

One approach is to simply stay in the flow and say something like, "Yes, that leg should be straight," or "Keep the elbows wrapped in," or whatever is the appropriate answer. If you find you don't know the answer (it could happen), you could say something like, "Wow, that is a good question! Let me find out!" This is always better than trying to fake it.

Remember, questions from people in class show a level of interest and commitment to learning. It's an attitude you want to encourage as much as possible. Even if you feel thrown off and you get a little flustered, simply suggest Child's Pose or Downward Facing Dog as a posture to get grounded again. If this is impossible due to where you're at in the sequence, hold the pose a bit longer while you gather yourself. Remember, it's okay in these situations to acknowledge you're a bit off in a graceful way. Even saying something like, Let's take a few breaths here to get connected," is an approach to give you 3-5 seconds to re-group.

A student asks you at the beginning of class to assist them in a particular pose.

Depending on your style of teaching, you may or may not provide hands-on assists during class. Teacher training programs sometimes only provide a short review on assisting so people graduate without having a real sense of how to assist students during class. However, if you've taken a specialty course in assisting or it was part of your training, you may be working assists into your class. Students can really get to love this and in fact, some may actually expect that you will assist them in certain postures.

When you assist a student, it is not only a reflection of your ability as a teacher but is also a reflection of your availability as a teacher. Your main role is to facilitate for the whole group, not for one individual student. This is part of what makes assisting while teaching an art. You need to keep the whole class moving forward, while you stop and work with one individual student. You also don't know how the student you're assisting will react and they may in fact, ask you some questions during the assist and you'll find yourself getting caught up in a quick conversation. It is for this reason that you should be clear when you approach a student as to your action to assist and still be able to keep an eye on the big picture.

Sometimes, during class, someone may ask you for an assist on the spot. Some students love to be assisted in a particular way in poses like Upward Bow or Pigeon. Depending on your availability, what else is going on in the room, your energy level and any other factors you need to consider, it may not be possible to assist the person. Rather than taking it personally or feeling badly, simply make eye contact with the student to acknowledge them and say something quietly, such as "Next time." Remember, it is not your obligation to assist anyone in a yoga pose. You don't need to say anything afterwards or apologize that you were not available for the assist. If you feel like you want to explain something to the person afterwards, you can but it may sound like you're making excuses. Remember, there are a lot of factors you are regularly working with when you teaching. Students won't know about these; they are only thinking about their own experience.

A student is spending much of the class lying down or in Child's Pose.

We always tell our students to take care of themselves while practicing. If we don't say it, it's certainly implied. We suggest certain things to help them do this like taking Child's Pose or other modifications. We may not literally suggest that they lie in Shavasana for much of the class but I have had a few situations where this has happened. Remember, students who rest during class are taking care of themselves. It isn't necessarily a reflection on you or your class; it has more to do with them. If you think they look dizzy, unsteady or ill, it might make sense to go over, gently place an arm on theirs and ask how they're doing. If they're in Child's Pose, sometimes a gentle assist is a nice acknowledgement. If you find a quiet time when they're resting, maybe a "How are you doing?" is a way to make a connection. But give them space to be where they are without making them feel guilty that they're taking care of themselves. Sometimes saying nothing is fine.

A student is in the middle of the room doing their own practice.

Sometimes, students are inspired to do variations of a posture that you are offering to the class. For instance, someone may take Prasarita Padottanasana (Wide Legged Forward Bend) into a Tripod Headstand. This is a logical extension of the pose and is easy to accommodate into the group practice. There may be other students, however, that use group classes as a way to fit in their own practice. They may, from the beginning of class, be doing a completely different sequence than you are offering and depending on where they placed themselves in the class, may be right in your line of sight as well as in full sight of other students trying to stay with the sequence you're offering.

For a newer teacher, or even a more experienced one, this can create quite a distraction. It can also be distracting to the people around the person. You will find that newer students will start to follow the one student or will be confused by what he or she is doing.

At this point, you need to make a call as to if you should ask the person to move their mat. This is not about you; it's about the group experience. If you find that the students around the person are watching and trying to mimic the person, take a moment when the class is in Downward Dog and quietly suggest to the student to move their mat to a private area in the room. Before you approach the person, make sure you have identified a spot so you can help them move their mat. This should be done with as little talking as possible. Remember to stay neutral. Also remember that if the person resists, let it be. There is no reason to make an issue over it. You are simply suggesting it. Your goal is to help the whole class and the student have space to do what they need to do, not to be right or to single out a person.

If you find that there are no extra spaces or there is no discrete way to ask the person to move (as in a class crowded with people), leave them be. As you are teaching, move around the room. Stick to the pace that works for the whole class.

After class, you may or may not wish to say something to the student about the fact that they practiced on their own. Remember, this is different from the scenario where someone is taking advanced variations in the same pose you have suggested; this is a student completely doing his or her own thing. If you choose to say something, approach from a observational perspective and say, "I noticed you were doing your own practice today." That might be it; just stating the observation. Or you could add, " Can you share your approach?" Remember, you don't want to put them on the defensive. Once you've said something, stop talking and let them speak. If you end up getting into a long conversation, it's probably gone too far. Your point is simply to bring awareness to the situation. If you find that this continues to happen, speak to the manager of the studio before approaching the student again if your next step is to be a bit more definitive with the student. Use the conversation with the manager to ensure you're on the same page and to check with someone else to be sure you get another opinion. If you do approach the student again because this continues to happen, leave them the option to come early and set up towards the back of the room. This is a nice compromise that allows the student to honor their practice and allows other students to take class without confusion or distraction.

A student tells you the studio is too hot.

Everyone has their own sense of what is appropriate temperature for a yoga class. Even in classes that are "Hot" yoga classes, there are differences between people as to what they may feel is an appropriate temperature. Most of the students that come to your class will abide by what is happening in the room and take steps to modify if they are too hot: rest, drink water, or step out of the room to help manage feeling too hot. However, some people may share with you their thoughts about the environment. It may come out as a comment or a request. Some may say, "Wow, it's really hot in here!" While others may say, "It's too hot. Can we turn it down?"

As a teacher, it's always your responsibility to tune into what the environment is like so you can be sure it's the right temperature for the experience. You need to make sure students have fresh oxygen, humidity and heat and the combination is appropriate given the class you are teaching. You must be looking at the class and watching them for signs of overheating or dizziness. You also need to look and notice if they are not sweating but are very red, which can be a sign that the room is too hot but there is no humidity.

If you have a student that comments out loud, you can say, " I hear you," or something to acknowledge that you heard what they said. Refrain from getting into a general discussion with the whole class; things like, "What do you all think?" only invites everyone to give their own opinion. This can become an unmanageable situation, as there is certainly no way to meet everyone's personal preference.

Take a moment with the student after class and check in with them.

Don't make apologies but ask them, "How are you doing?" This will most likely turn into a conversation about the room temperature. Give them strategies to manage the heat. Hear what they are saying. Don't contribute to the concerns and turn it into a complaint session. Give them information about what you're looking at in terms of the room and what you expect the room to be like for students. Ultimately, this person needs to decide if this class is the right one for them.

A student passes out.

It's critical that as yoga teacher, you are First Aid and CPR Certified so if you are faced with a medical emergency, you can confidently take charge. In some cases, you may be the only studio employee onsite; in other cases, there may be an assistant, manager or front desk associate there as well. Either way, your role is to immediately go to the student ("check the scene, check the victim"- the first steps of CPR) and specifically ask another student to "Call 911 and report back to me." Beyond that, additional specific and appropriate CPR/first aid guidelines should be carried out.

Remember, as the teacher of the class, your main role is to stay with the injured person. It is not to run outside the room to call or wait for emergency personnel. Anyone else in the room can do that and can run to get another studio employee (if there is one available).

These circumstances, unfortunately, are opportunities for you to practice what you teach: staying calm in the moment is a function of deep breathing, focusing and staying connected to your body.

Closing Summary

The reality is that no matter how prepared you are, there will always be something that comes up in class that you didn't expect. As you get more experienced, this will be less of an issue and you will be less thrown by these curve balls as they come up. When you're newer, it can be distracting and can throw you off course. Always keep in mind that as long as you keep the idea of "being of service" in mind, any reaction you have will be softened. This will help you as well to keep centered and in the body as you manage whatever arises.

Chapter 14

How to Build a Class Around a Theme

Focus

I've shared in a few different chapters the idea that as a new teacher, it's helpful to have a standard sequence that you provide when teaching. This allows you to focus less on what you're going to offer and more on what's actually happening in the room. Teaching a different sequence every time, or even every week can be quite unsettling for a new teacher because you're left wondering what's next to offer in the sequence. Even if you practice it before several times, the reality is once you're in front of the class you will inevitably forget and have to re-group.

For that reason, as a new teacher, having a standard theme is a great idea because it allows you to focus more on the students, how your instruction is being received, assisting and speaking from the heart. It removes a big obstacle to one of the primary reasons you're there: to connect with your students. It does this by taking you out of your head and allowing you to be really present.

Overall Considerations

Once you've been teaching for a while (I would suggest at least 2-3 times per week for a few years), you may want to stray from the standard sequence. Once you do that though, it can be helpful to have a template that you use to "contain" your classes. In other words, you need something to "bind together" all the poses you offer. An ideal thing to provide this structure is a theme. Themes can be physical or they can be intellectual or spiritual; you can also blend one physical theme and another one that is more intellectual into one class. Providing a theme in a class is a way to help students see the similarities between poses or to perhaps understand how themes from yoga practice can translate into other areas of their life. Let's take a look at some of the themes that you can bring into class.

Physical Themes

Grounding/Steadiness: This theme could be emphasized by staying with essential, basic poses and focusing on the alignment, along with calling attention to the straight lines present in each pose. Props can be used to create a physical experience of steadiness as well as comments about how the foundation we create in poses can create a sense of steadiness in our lives.

Opening/External rotation: Poses that emphasize external rotation through the hips and shoulders illustrate this theme on a physical level. Speaking to the expansion one feels when in these kinds of postures brings the theme to a higher level. These poses can also bring students into the opposite direction (opening the chest versus hunching) and this is the opposite shape from what they are in for most of the day.

Balancing: These poses can bring up a great deal of frustration for students as they fall out of a pose. Offering this as a theme allows you to challenge their sense of balance, helps them develop stronger legs and also examine how these poses push their buttons.

Learning/Discovery: You may choose to go into class with the intention to explain something in more detail. It could be something that is done all the time in class and you want to be sure students understand the alignment. An example of this would be the proper way to move from High to Low Push Up. This theme speaks to the student's ability to stay open to learning, even if they think they already know how to do the pose. Testing their ability to be a "beginner" is part of sharing how "beginner's mind" is critical to being present and open as a yoga student.

Relaxing/Centering: Presenting poses that are more restorative in nature gives the students a chance to slow down and notice how their body feels. In the warm summer months, this can have a cooling effect. Even if you teach heated classes, you can use a slightly slower pace to create a more restful feel to the practice. Speak to creating a strong foundation, working from the "center out," and encouraging students to rest when they need to do so.

Twisting/Rinsing: Focusing the practice on twists, both in standing postures as well as those on the floor can be a tremendous release. Using this as a theme allows you the chance to speak to how the breath fuels the twist and how twists aid digestion and strengthen the core. The physical movement of twisting brings up the idea of getting rid of what is not needed in the body and relieving stress.

Breathing/Meditating: Starting class with a seated meditation will allow this theme to work its way nicely into the class. You can support the idea of creating a meditative space by sticking to an essential sequence and keeping your verbal instruction focused, brief but effective. This theme works well when people seem to be very stressed, you have a restorative class or something has happened in the local, regional or national arena that is creating stress and pain for the public. Living in the Northeast where our winters can be long and cold, it's a great way to help people manage the stress of a long winter.

Strengthening/Challenging: Focusing on poses to strengthen can give people a feeling of accomplishment and stability. Including poses like Warrior 1 and 2, Side Plank, Crow, Half Moon as well as including abdominal work can help your students build strength and stamina. Speaking to their sense of "inner strength" can help them to acknowledge that they may be stronger than they think.

Holding/Working with resistance: While this can be a tough theme to bring into class and stay committed to as a teacher, it can be a great way to challenge your students to relax in their bodies while receiving strong feedback at the same time. This theme would work well in a restorative class but can also work in a flow class if you hold the poses towards the end of class longer and focus on hip openers.

Listening to intuition: This theme is wonderful for encouraging people to listen to their own sense of what works for them in each pose. You could bring this up as a theme by speaking to it at the beginning of class. You could use very essential instruction to give students' ample space and room to move into each pose on their own. Once you've taught one or two Sun Salutation A's and B's, allow students to move through the sequences on their own as this is a great way to have them listen to their breath and their own inner guidance.

Themes inspired by challenges we may face

You injured yourself, on or off the mat, and need to modify your yoga practice: This is such a great theme to bring into class because everyone will experience injuries at some point. Working on the mat within our capabilities on that particular day is part of a healthy yoga practice. You could use your personal experience with injury to suggest more modifications to your students, to bring in the idea of the first Yama, ahimsa (one of the 8 Limbs of Yoga), which speaks to non-harming behaviors or to suggest using props. You could also speak to pushing yourself or losing the integrity of the postures because of an ideal you're holding out there around how the poses "should" look rather than how they can be expressed in your body. You could also bring into class the idea of practicing with compassion, not as "way out" but more as a way to respect your body.

You recently ended a romantic relationship: Yoga is a heart-opening practice, both on a physical and emotional level. Many of the poses ask you to roll your shoulders back and open your chest. Poses like Upward Facing Dog, Camel, Fish and Upward Bow all literally "open your heart." For someone going through a break-up, these poses can express the very feelings they're trying to avoid and you may be experiencing the same thing. Themes that can come from this experience can be around the idea of letting feelings and sensations arise in your body in each pose without judging them, having faith that what you want in your life and the practice will show up, or being true to yourself, both on and off the mat (something you may doubt after a break-up). You could also share the idea of practicing with compassion as way to help you be more compassionate to yourself in other areas of your life.

You recently experienced the death of someone in your life: Loss is part of life but a painful part. We all experience it in the form of losing someone we love, losing a pet, losing a friend. You could speak about the transient nature of things, appreciating what you have in the moment or the power of being present as a way to feel some relief from the challenges you may be facing in your life. You could speak to emotions that might be arising and having the courage to face them, rather than stuffing them down. You could talk about how yoga provides us with strength, not only in our bodies, but also in our hearts and minds, so that we can withstand the ups and downs of life.

You're struggling with issues at work that are creating frustration and anger: When we struggle in a situation, we need to step back and find space, so we can gain perspective. This is a great theme for yoga because you can speak to how different poses give us a different point of view, literally, and this can help you gain new perspective. You can also talk about the idea of being right versus being at peace and how while you may be right, trying to prove that to others can create stress. You could speak to being frustrated in a pose and using the breath to find relief.

You're having a hard time making ends meet financially: When we're struggling to make ends meet, we can see the world from the view of what we don't have, rather than what we do. This can translate to our approach to our bodies and our yoga practice. We can focus on what appears to be lacking in our practice or we can be grateful that we're on the mat, even if we practice yoga from a restorative perspective or spend 15 minutes in Child's Pose, breathing deeply.

Here are a few examples of physical themes you can bring into your classes and examples of what you could offer that would reinforce the theme:

Breath

There is nothing more central to yoga than the breath. Weaving a theme around the breath can give students a powerful tool they can use in any class.

- Start sitting on a block and demonstrate Ujjayi breath
- As you move through the opening Sun Salutations, shift the last 3 Sun A's and Sun B's into "breath only" cueing. This can be a powerful way to show how breathing and moving work together
- Share information about the relaxation response, to help them see the connection on an organic level between deep breathing and feeling relaxed in the body
- End class with some simple pranayama breathing exercises

Uddiyana Bandha

The technique of drawing the abdomen in towards the spine is a powerful one for yoga practice as it helps students create "lift" in the body. This "lift" can be used for several things, including jumping forward to the front of the mat, jumping into Low push up (from halfway lift) in Sun Salutations, Crow pose and other arm balances.

- Start students standing and demonstrate Uddiyana Bandha
- As you move them through Sun Salutation A and B, introduce "jumping forward" from Down Dog to the front of mat
- Demonstrate jumping from halfway lift to Low push up and offer 3 more Sun Salutations with the option to jump into Low push up
- Use poses like Boat and Crow to emphasize how the core lock stabilizes the body

Setting a firm foundation

Setting a firm foundation in each pose is essential for helping students feel stable as well as giving the body the support it needs to take several twisting postures, like Twisting Crescent Lunge and Twisting Triangle.

- Start students in Mountain Pose. Ask them to notice the stacking of joints and the feeling of stability in the body
- Instruct on the use of blocks to create a firm foundation and encourage students to bring their hand to the inside of the foot as they take twists to try a more stable foundation
- Use poses like Upward Dog, Cat/Cow sequence, Warrior 1 and Bridge to emphasize how stacking the joints creates a firm foundation
- Use balancing poses like Tree, Dancer's and Eagle to reinforce the importance of foundation to balancing the whole body

Using the muscles of the middle and upper back to open the chest

Many people come to yoga with little awareness of the muscles of the middle and upper back. Spending much of our days hunched over computers and Smart Phones, we feel the effects of a collapsed chest but often lack the knowledge about how to reverse this condition. Yoga gives us many poses and sequence that help us open our chests, which for many, can be an emotional experience as well as they begin to open their heart center.

- Start students in Mountain Pose. Have them close their eyes and instruct to draw the shoulder blades in and down. Ask them to notice how these movements open the heart center
- In Upward Dog, emphasize the movement of the shoulders "back" and "down" making special note of how the neck is relaxed
- Use poses like Dancer's, Camel, Locust, Bow, Bridge, Upward Bow and Fish to emphasize using the middle to upper back to open the heart center
- In Shavasana, have student place on hand on their heart to help them connect to physical sensations in the body

Closing Summary

Once you start exploring different themes to weave into your classes and bind the poses together, you can really begin to challenge yourself as a teacher. This is not to say that there are not challenges inherent in sticking to a traditional sequence from class to class but there is an interesting challenge you face when you start with a theme and then build a class around the theme. Once you've been teaching for some time, you may be looking for new ways to grow and expand not only your teaching expertise but ways to bring different poses into your teaching. Building a class around a theme is a great way to do both things.

Chapter 15

How to Build Connection with Your Students

Focus

You can strive to teach challenging, fun and inspiring yoga classes but without connection to your students, the class may fall flat. Sometimes you'll teach a class and your head will be filled with imaginary feedback ("She looks really annoyed; she must be hating this class" or "He looks like he's really struggling; he'll never come back"); other times you'll feel like the class and you are working together as one synchronized unit.

Building connection can be hard but is one of the most important factors in teaching classes where your students feel supported, seen and acknowledged. For you as a teacher, teaching classes where you're building connection is challenging but rewarding in a way that is almost indescribable. So, how do you build connection? There are definitely some things that you can do that will help to create the right conditions for connection but ultimately, you have to trust that connection will happen when the overall conditions are right for it to show up. Some of this can't really be "taught" per se, but there is definitely the possibility of connection when you do certain things. Remember, you can never force connection; it really just needs to show up on it's own.

Overall Considerations

Giving alignment tips that specifically address what you see: If you notice someone has a knee beyond a heel in Warrior 1, suggest they stack their joints. If you notice someone's face is completely scrunched up in Bow, suggest relaxing the face. Chances are the suggestion will be helpful to more than one student and the individual student will feel acknowledged.

Sharing from your heart: When you share your own thoughts, not to speak about yourself but to inspire and educate, you build connection.

People will sense if you're trying to be someone you're not. When you share from the heart, you inspire your students and show yourself. Through this action, you build connection.

Allowing for space and silence: When most people come to yoga class, they are tired, over-stimulated and stressed. They are looking for exercise, maybe they're passionate about yoga or maybe they're new to the practice but in any event, they most likely are not looking to be "talked at" for an hour. When you give them some space to hear their breath and quiet their mind, you're giving them a chance to build connection with you, with themselves and also with the class as a whole.

Assisting students: Many students, as much as you are creative with what you say, have a hard time understanding alignment cues. When you approach a student to assist them in a pose (with a goal of compassion and understanding, not just correction), you build a connection with that student by showing them your goal is to help them understand and experience yoga.

Disconnection can happen when:

You have a set agenda for what you'll teach despite what's right in front of you: It's great to have a plan, a set flow and even a plan for what you'll read after class (if you do that kind of thing). But when you go into a class full of people, not knowing who will be there, how they'll be and charge ahead with your agenda, that can be a disconnect from what's happening in the moment. Have your plan but be ready to change it if you need to. This can be something along the lines of slowing it down, picking up the pace, dropping some poses or adding more personal instruction.

Teaching with your back to the class, from the back of the room or practicing with the class: This is a tricky one because in many instances, any of these techniques can be very effective and useful so I should add that disclaimer. But, in general, once you can't see your students, it's can be a challenge to build connection.

You go on autopilot, trying to cram in as much instruction around alignment as possible: We want our students to "get it" but once we start overwhelming them with alignment tips, they check out. They're already overwhelmed when they get there and throwing 10 tips in long sentences at them while in Warrior 1 can be too much.

Telling your students what they should feel: We teach from our own experience of yoga in our body, along with the understanding, as a teacher, of the intention of the pose. Downward Facing Dog focuses on stretching the spine and feeling length in the hamstrings but it's common for many students to feel pain in their hands, rounding in the back and stress in the legs. When we state: "Feel length in your spine" we assume they can get there. Instead, we can give alignment tips to help them get there and suggest what they might feel. This can be even more challenging when we speak to the relaxation they might feel. For instance, in Shavasana, it's assumed that students will be able to "relax in their bodies" but for some students, they may find themselves anxious or their minds still going furiously. Rather than telling them to "Relax" try suggesting they breathe, open the chest and close their eyes. Beyond that, the rest can be up to them.

Closing Summary

Ultimately, one of the central ideas of yoga teaching is for you to create the ideal conditions under which students are able to connect to the present and their bodies. We've reviewed a number of ways you can do this but ultimately, it is up to the student. However, through these techniques and others you try, with variable success, you will find that there are great opportunities for you to create these conditions for your students. Through connection, their experience in your classes can take on an additional depth beyond the physical and help you develop a regular relationship with a number of students who will want to regularly attend your classes. Again, this can't be something we force but it is certainly an angle of teaching we must consider.

Chapter 16

How to Bring Themes of Classic Yoga Philosophy into Your Teaching

Focus

When we teach yoga poses, or the asanas, we must recognize that we are only presenting one aspect of yoga as a practice. Asana, as one limb of the Eight-Limb Path of Yoga, is just one component of the whole system of yoga and is the most commonly accessed part of yoga itself. However, as teachers, it's helpful to integrate other aspects of the practice of yoga into our teaching. In this way, we can educate students about the other aspects of the practice that are often overlooked. However, the challenge is to keep the class moving, avoid overwhelming students and avoid sounding like we're preaching. We also need to know the other limbs of the practice and a contemporary and understandable way to present them to students.

Overall Considerations

The Mind/Body Connection

While we don't always bring into class themes inspired by classic yoga philosophy, nor are many of our students familiar with them, most everyone is familiar with the concept of the "mind/body connection." This term refers to the idea that how one feels in the body can impact the mind and of course, how one's thoughts impact the body. We're probably familiar with stories of how patients with cancer improved their physical condition through the use of yoga and meditation and how practicing yoga helps people suffering from depression. This idea that our thoughts can alter our physical condition gives us a springboard from which to introduce the other concepts of yoga that are outside of the asana. The other aspects of yoga practice cover aspects of the mind and ways of being that are all centered around living in balance, living in a way aligned to certain principles, staying present and internally focused.

The Eight Limbs and Applying the Concepts to Your Classes

The Eight Limbed Path outlined in Patanjali's Yoga Sutras, gives us an framework for approaching life and carrying ourselves in such a way as to respect others, respect ourselves and manage the variability in the mind that occurs when we waver between distraction and concentration, and all the stages in between. It starts with a concept called the Yamas, known as the moral restraints. The Five Moral Restraints are:

- Ahimsa - nonviolence
- Satya - truthfulness
- Asteya - nonstealing
- Brahmacharya - moderation
- Aparigraha - nonhoarding

Let's go through these one by one and look at themes we can apply to teaching.

Ahimsa: this means non-violence in both action and thought. We could refer to themes around being mindful in our movements, watching for alignment errors that create injury, watching our movements for times when we're pushing too hard and end up sitting in our joints. We could refer to thoughts we might be having that are fueled by punishing ourselves for not practicing regularly rather than showing compassion and acknowledging the good work we're already doing by just showing up on the mat. We could refer to words we use when speaking about our lives or our practice and things we say that show disrespect to ourselves and others.

Satya: this refers to being truthful and speaking the truth. While this might be a stretch to apply to practice as we're not speaking, remember that "truth" in this context can also apply to being truthful with ourselves. What better way to illustrate this than the concept of modifying a yoga practice. When we modify a pose, we're being truthful with ourselves about what we believe is within our capabilities at the time. It's also a way to be truthful about the impact of injuries on our body and acknowldge that modifying is a way for us to still practice but with consideration of our injury.

Asteya: The literal translation for this yama is "nonstealing" or the idea of refraining from taking that which is not your own. While you may think of this and wonder how it could apply to yoga, if you think of the concept of "stealing" and think of it in the context of stealing from yourself (good thoughts, time to do yoga) or taking more than you need (of yoga props, space in the studio) you can start to see how you could use themes of asteya in teaching.

Brahmacharya: the literal translation of this yama means "celibacy" but could be thought of as the concept of being faithful to yourself and someone with whom you're in a relationship. Themes like being faithful to your practice, while not a direct translation, might be another way to bring this into class. Keep in mind however, that something along these lines might not be a topic to raise in class due to student sensitivity around sexuality.

Aparigraha: This is the concept of non-possessiveness or the concept of self-restraint. While we can think of this in terms of possessing material things there are other themes we can bring into class that have to do with letting go of things we don't need that are not material: things like negative thoughts, jealously, anger, self-hatred or judgment. These all make wonderful themes for class because there is much we hold onto as students of yoga that gets in the way of our "naturalness." These things involve thoughts of self-doubt or feelings of lack of self-worth, especially when it comes to our abilities around yoga practice itself. Releasing these feelings, inspired by the theme of "aparigraha" can free us up to move more gracefully and with more compassion for our body.

After the Yamas come the Niyamas, or the Five Spiritual Observances. They are:

- Sauca: Purity
- Santosha: Contentment
- Tapas: Zeal, Austerity
- Svadhyaya: Self-study
- Ishvara-Pranidhana: Devotion to a higher power

Let's go through these characteristics one by one and see how we can apply them to our teaching.

Sauca: Literally translated, this means "cleanliness." Of course, we can take that literally and think about the cleanliness of our bodies and minds. We can bring to the awareness of our students the idea that be grateful, not using inappropriate language or even classifying our practice as "good" or "bad" attaches a label to it that can imply judgment. Keeping our speech "clean" is as important as taking a shower or brushing our teeth. The other aspect of cleanliness has to do with how we approach our practice area. We can be respectful of ourselves and others by setting up a clean space in an orderly way in the studio. We can be mindful of others around us by keeping our props close by and not stepping on others' mats. We can also be courteous and put away our props neatly so they are neat for the next students that need them.

Santosha: This refers to the feeling of contentment, something that gets harder and harder to have in our contemporary society. Students come to yoga wanting their body to look like someone else's, want the cool yoga clothes of the person next to them or perhaps want to do a pose that they cannot do. All of this "wanting for what we don't have" can lead to a feeling of lack or discontent with the way things are. We can help our students recognize that having a lack of attachment to material things or even ways of being can help us find more peace with the way things are right now. This can lead to a feeling of contentment, even if it means we are still striving to be better, grow more and work towards certain poses.

Tapas: Tapas comes from the Sanskit verb "tap" which means "to burn". When we think about "burning energy" in yoga, we can refer to it as a discipline that is fueled by commitment and a energy of fire that refuses to be extinguished. We can apply this concept to our teaching by sharing with students the importance of staying committed to the practice without being attached to the results. We may be excited to see results in the form of changes in our bodies and our ability to do certain poses. But one of the challenges is to stay on track even when those changes aren't coming as fast and furious as they often do at the start of our practice. We can also apply this concept to our careers and how we find the strength to continue in a career when things are not going well.

Svadhyaya: Literally translated, this means to "recite or repeat or rehearse to oneself." As students of yoga, we see this repetition in the mantras we chant before and after class. We might also see this in mantras or sayings we repeat to ourselves to carry us through a tough practice or a time time in our lives. The other aspect of Svadhyaya is found in the concept of the study of scripture. Pantanjali referred to the Yoga Sutras, but in contemporary society, we could consider this studying anything that is important to us from the perspective of personal or career growth. We could even refer to the study of yoga and yoga philosophy as a way to live this aspect of the practice.

Ishvara-Pranidhana: This means, " surrendering to a higher source," and while this might seem like a religious reference, it gives us a chance as teachers to help students appreciate the idea that all is not within their control and peace can be found when we give up trying to control it all. Certainly for someone whose personal belief system involves honoring a higher source, this could come into play as well but there is also the concept of surrender. We surrender control on our mat by making peace with things the way they are in the moment.

Now that we've gone through the components of the first two Limbs of Yoga, the Yamas and the Niyamas, we can move onto the other 6 limbs of yoga.

The third limb is Asana. This refers to the postures we do. As I said at the beginning of this chapter, this is the most commonly experienced limb of Yoga as this is what most students do and what most studios offer. While meditation, which we will get to later in this discussion, is a huge part of the practice, the main aspect that students can relate to are the poses themselves. As teachers, we can help our students realize that this is only one aspect of yoga and the more we can open our minds to other aspects, the more depth our practice will have, both on and off the mat.

The fourth Limb of Yoga is Pranayama. This refers to mindful breathing and the many ways to do this. As teachers, we can refer to "Ujjayi breathing" throughout class and show our students how to do it. This is only one breathing technique and we can expand our students' knowledge of Pranayama by sharing different styles of breathing. We can also speak to shifting awareness from the outside to the inside by bringing more awareness to our breath and can help students recognize how focusing on the breath has a calming effect on the body and mind.

The fifth Limb of Yoga is Pratyahara, which is known as a "turning inward." When you look at the next four limbs, you can see a progression from focusing on the outside to focusing more on the inside in a deeper way that even just through the practice of pranayama. This idea of turning inward speaks to our choice to withdraw from what is happening around us and focus instead on ourselves. This is seen most commonly at the end of yoga class, when we ask students to rest in Shavasana. In this relaxed state, students are aware of their external surroundings but they choose to stay focused on the internal so they can rest their bodies and minds and seal in the goodness of their practice. We can encourage people to take this concept with them as they go out into their lives as well. Students come to class overwhelmed with the stimulation they get through exposure to people, media and computers all day. This can get overwhelming at times and can bring up feelings of overwhelm, depression and even anger. Calling on the concept of Pratyahara in these times can help people to decompress and put themselves first.

The next limb is Dharana. When we are able to sustain our concentration, this is known as Dharana. Also referred to as "holding focus," we can see how easily this translates to yoga teaching and practice. While hard to do, we encourage our students all the time to try to keep their focus on one fixed point so as to discourage distractions. We can encourage students to stay with the practice, through the good times and the not so great times, to train the mind to be able to stay focused on one point. There are so many opportunities for distraction both on the mat and off, and as we bring this concept into our classes, we help our students see that they can train their minds to be more focused, despite all that is going on around them.

The seventh limb of yoga is Dhyana. As we move from sustained concentration deeper into the sense of the Self, we begin to move into the 7th Limb of Yoga called Dhyana or "meditation." As teachers, we can let our students know that this limb is the next phase on the final path from Dharana (above) to Samadhi (final Limb of Yoga). This takes the concept of concentration and moves it beyond the withdrawl of the senses and focusing on one thing to going even deeper into a meditative state.

The eighth or final Limb of Yoga is known as "the Union of the Self with the Object of Meditation." Some refer to it as reaching a stage of Enlightenment. While this might seem a lofty state to even raise in our culture of self-centeredness and immediacy, it's a great way to help students recognize that with surrender, an ability to be content with the way things are and a commitment to practice both yoga and meditation, we can move towards a state of greater inner peace. This can start with how we approach our practice, can grow by building these other aspects of Yoga into our lives and our practice and can help us see how there is a continuum of movement towards a state where we can find great contentment.

Closing Summary

There are many ways we can bring these foundations of the practice of yoga into our classes. As always, sharing from the heart and speaking truthfully but essentially as well will keep the information expanding the knowledge of the student without making it about the teacher. As teachers, we need to look for opportunities to expand students' knowledge about yoga from the poses to the other aspects of the practice, not only so that they can understand it is a multi-dimensional practice but so that they may work towards greater peace in their lives.

Chapter 17

How to Let Your True Nature Come Through in Your Teaching

Focus

As teachers, we use the poses as the way to build strength and flexibility in the body. Although the poses are defined in a certain way in terms of alignment, they're expressed differently depending on the teacher. A good example of this is the request for students to reach their arms up above their head. You can ask them in any number of ways and use different tone, pace, words, volume and inflection in the voice to create the action. But every teacher will sound differently and each student will perceive what they hear differently, depending on the teacher. This is, in large part, due to the different way each teacher expresses his or herself through the practice of teaching yoga.

One of the challenges we have is finding the right balance between sharing enough so that we're real, spontaneous and approachable but not over-sharing to the point where we start to become a distraction to the students. How we do this is an art and can be one of the hallmarks to allow us to distinguish ourselves as teachers. So how much is too much and what should you share and how?

There are several different ways to approach this:

Share something about yourself but make use of a story highlighting a general theme that might be common to all.

These themes below are similar to the themes that I suggested in the earlier chapter on How to Build Your Class Around a Theme. You could share a general theme about loss, fueled by your recent experience of breaking up a relationship. You might talk about managing injuries, modifying or taking care of yourself, based on your recent experience with an injury. You might have experienced a loss in your life and could share the idea of being appreciative about what we have.

Use **humor**

One of the best pieces of advice one of my teachers, Baron Baptiste, gave me was the advice to "keep things light." While this doesn't mean to ignore alignment errors or to be casual about your approach to teaching, it does mean to keep "lightness" to your approach so that people feel comfortable and free of judgment and pressure to conform to a certain standard. Using humor is one way to create this kind of environment and while it doesn't mean you're cracking jokes non-stop, it might mean you laugh at yourself if you trip over your words or could mean you mention a funny article or something that you think would make people laugh. It could even mean you tell a bad joke just to get people to loosen up a bit.

Comedians will tell you it's one of the loneliest jobs in the world, that of joke telling, because you're hoping for a laugh and taking a risk because the joke could fall flat on its face. As a yoga teacher, the stakes aren't as high but it could be just as risky to you to attempt to make people laugh for fear that they won't. It's usually these fear-based situations that are the perfect chance for you to take the risk and share of yourself. What's the worst-case scenario? You'd have given it a try and it didn't work. But in the process, you shared of yourself and many of your students will appreciate you for that.

Use examples from teaching to illustrate a point

There are always themes we can use as teaching tools and they come up all the time. If we're awake and aware, we can keep these in mind and use them in our teaching to reinforce a point or to help people see that their questions are not unique. Many times, people won't ask a question because they think they'll look silly or appear to be a new student. So, the more you can bring up examples, you'll reassure your students that they're not the only ones to have the question and can reinforce proper action. In your explanation, there's an opportunity to share of yourself and step outside the general standard of giving physical instruction.

Use general themes that are based in yoga practice

We talked about these themes in Chapter 14. Working with these themes can be a way to share a little bit of yourself as you work these themes into class.

Smile as you teach

One of the greatest tools we have for self-expression is to smile. While this isn't something that you'd do non-stop, as opportunities arise where there's a genuine expression of happiness or connection, use facial expressions to connect, share of your personality and heart and show people you're real.

Share what has worked for you and why you love the practice

While you've probably heard " Yoga has changed my life" a hundred times, either by reading it in a teacher's biography or article or hearing it in class, underlying this general statement are a number of benefits to yoga that make perfect fodder to share with class. If you can personalize the sharing of this information in some way, it allows you to share from your heart, while providing the class with basic themes that they can use to assist them with their own practice.

Self-Assessment and Exploration Tools to get at themes for your teaching

If you're feeling a bit stuck around themes you could bring into your classes or ways you can share beyond the poses, here are some general questions to ask yourself to get the creative thoughts flowing:

Why do you love yoga?

What benefits has yoga brought to you?

How has yoga helped you through a difficult time?

What are the challenges you face in your yoga practice?

What's the funniest thing that happened to you in a yoga pose?

How do you manage frustration on the mat?

Have you ever cried during practice and what triggered the emotion?

Do you have a favorite yoga pose and one you don't like and why?

Closing Summary

One of the hardest things for people to do is to step outside the basics of teaching the poses and share from the heart. For others, they might have such an easy time, that their classes are filled with personal stories, teaching anecdotes and themes from yoga. Finding a teacher with whom you can connect will be based in large part on how their style of sharing connects with yours but can be one of the biggest factors for you as a teacher in terms of building your name, your unique style and distinguishing factors.

Chapter 18

Facing your Fears as a Yoga Teacher

Focus

As a yoga teacher, one aspect of our job is to help people face their fears. We do it by challenging students to stay in a pose, face the poses they prefer to avoid, and breathe deeply through a complex sequence.

But what about us as teachers? What fears might we have that need to be brought to light? We don't often talk to each other about our fears. We stay positive and share our success stories: the sold out workshop, the connection we made with a student, the success of our first retreat. But inside, we all have them. Our personal list might be filled with thoughts around body image, presentation, personal style, knowledge and experience. But to deny we have them is to avoid finding healthy ways to work through them. When we avoid working through them, they remain as barriers to our growth.

Here are a few that come to my mind, through my own personal experience.

Overall Considerations

That teacher is better than me.

Have you ever taken a class and thought that you're inadequate on some level as a teacher? It's easy to compare our teaching to others. We can do it by taking someone's class, we can do it through watching what they're up to on social media and making assumptions about the quality of their teaching. We can do it by overhearing what others say about teachers they love.

Comparisons work to do two important things: they can help secure us in the knowledge that we're teaching in a way that is consistent with our sense of self and they can challenge us to push our boundaries.

The teacher that you feel knows more about yoga philosophy can be the catalyst to you taking a course on the Sutras; the one that teaches a popular heated yoga class can confirm for you that this style is just not your thing. Taking a class as a student is not an objective experience; there is no way one can say, "This is the right way to teach and this is the wrong way." Be responsible and accountable to know the essentials around teaching but find your own way of expressing it.

That teacher has bigger classes than me.

Did you ever see the posts on Facebook where teachers note how many students were in their class and wonder if you'll ever have a packed room? There are many angles to consider: time of class, location, prior experience of the teacher or whether or not he or she has an existing following.

There are steps we can take as teachers to promote our classes. These should be taken to generate interest and attendance. But at the end of the day, the ultimate decision is the student's. Your job is to do your absolute best in your teaching and be willing to the take the risk to share of yourself. The more you do, the more you will create connections with your students and build your classes. This kind of fear is circular and is a slippery slope to self-doubt that will plague you for your teaching career if not faced immediately. Do what you can do to control what you can and have faith and believe in yourself, no matter what the outcome. Also have the strength to be open to feedback and exploring what might be missing.

If I were to host my own retreat or workshop, I won't have enough people to fill it.

Have you ever thought you'd like to do a retreat or host a workshop but you stop out of fear that no one will show up? Or that you'll have to cancel it due to not meeting the minimum number of people necessary to hold the event?

There definitely are logistics to hosting your own workshops and retreats. It should be part of your research that you understand what the minimum number of attendees is and that you plan for it. This minimum attendance and subsequent revenue should take into consideration the factors important to you: the time to plan and execute the event, travel time, lost revenue from getting coverage for your regular classes, your overall experience. You must take marketing steps targeted at generating sufficient interest to meet the minimum. It might mean setting an up-front minimum with the host studio or retreat center so you plan for the possibility of canceling the event. Or you may decide it's worth it to hold the event regardless of how many people attend because it's great experience for you.

Once that's done, put your energy into marketing the event, talking it up, sharing it with the students in your classes and posting about it on your social media pages. If it needs to be canceled due to low attendance, take time to review what happened. Did you have people sign up and cancel a few days before? Why did they cancel? Did you schedule the event on a holiday weekend? What can you learn from others who have hosted events that have worked?

Even if you don't hold the event, was it a failure? It's only a failure if you avoid trying and putting yourself out there out of fear.

I don't think they like this class.

Ah, the thoughts we think while we teach. We may look at the class and try to figure out what students are thinking based on how they look. We try to read their minds by looking at their appearance. Our brain runs in different directions as we adjust what we're doing based on the assumed feedback we're receiving or we ignore that feedback and stay on our original path. The energy to do all of this is exhausting.

We must teach in a way that is natural to us. As soon as we start to imitate, emulate or do what we think the students want, we're in trouble. That's an image that takes an incredible amount of energy to uphold and we will never be able to present a class that meets everyone's idea of a perfect experience. It's completely understandable to take on some of the intonation or phrasing of teachers with whom we've trained; but eventually, if not really immediately, we need to find our own voice. While some of the technique may be borrowed, our expression should be our own. If not, how will anyone have a sense of who you are and have an opportunity to bond with you? When you hide behind someone else's way of being, you're robbing your students of the chance to see who you really are.

The reality is there is no "right" way to teach. While there may be correct ways to approach things from a technical perspective, outside of that aspect of teaching, our responsibility lies in teaching from our hearts. Our goal of "how can I help?" as Deepak Chopra would say, always puts us in the right frame of mind to be of service. And this is our ultimate role as a teacher.

I don't know enough about yoga to be a teacher.

There is much to learn, understand and know to be a yoga teacher. The path to learning is endless and filled with both the hands-on aspects of teaching as well as the academic aspects of learning about yoga history, philosophy, anatomy and the myriad of other aspects of teaching.

Along with what you must learn to teach, there's the aspect of personal expression. What you learn will be filtered through your own sense of expression and personal presentation. The reality is there isn't a way that you can know everything. Some teachers will be heavier on asana; some teachers will be heavier on philosophy or anatomy. We need to find a blend that feels right to us. If you feel there are areas where you are lacking in knowledge, it's critical that you do what's needed to seek out the missing data. Also, as a teacher, be open to saying, "I don't know" when asked a question and don't know the answer (then go and research it to find out). The best thing we can offer our students is our commitment to do our best.

Fear is at the heart of every obstacle we face as teachers. It's the same fear that actors speak of when they receive awards; it's the fear athletes speak of when they win championships. Pretending it's not there is to do ourselves a disservice to our own growth. Assuming that you're the only one that has them is wrong. It's through the path of trying and doing our best that we will grow rich in experience and this experience will only enrich what we can offer our classes as we teach.

Closing Summary

Fear, while it can be debilitating, can also lead to exhilaration when we conquer it. This doesn't always require overcoming a huge obstacle; it could be fear of teaching a new pose or fear of telling a short story relevant to the theme of the class. The common approach in all of these scenarios is to face fear and do it anyway!

Chapter 19

Teaching Yoga to Beginners

Focus

In any yoga teacher's career, you will run into people that have never practiced yoga before. Some teachers will focus primarily on teaching beginners; other teachers will run into beginners in their open level classes. It's inevitable and it's one of the wonderful things about teaching yoga. When you meet a new student, it's a magical time for them (even if they don't realize it). Your ability to communicate clearly and effectively, as well as show them compassion and support, can make the difference between their continuing with yoga or bailing out after their first class.

In order to maximize the initial experience of the student, there are a few variables to consider:

- The practice itself; poses and sequence
- The physical space and where the student is in the room
- Props available to you and the student
- The language used in teaching
- Assisting provided

Let's start with some general, overall considerations.

Overall Considerations

Keep your language essential and focused on the desired actions you want to see in their bodies. Say exactly what you want them to do, with as little additional explanation as possible. Use action words like "press," "lift" and "stretch" (see also my prior Chapter titled, "Effective Language for Yoga Teaching")' and only occasionally use the more artistic, creative descriptions that might be used in a class with more experienced students.

Keep your sequencing consistent from class to class. This is especially true if you teach a Beginner's class. Students will learn from repetition and their bodies and minds will remember more from class to class if you continue to reinforce the same sequence. This consistent presentation will also help them, over time, to start to shift from thinking about each movement to connecting more to a meditative feeling. As more experienced practitioners, we know that this is possible, but it's much harder when you don't know how to do each pose and you'll only make it harder for them if you switch up the sequence each week.

Ask them questions about their experience. I like to open my Beginner's Classes with a breakdown of a pose or asking students before class, "What pose really challenges you?" or any other specific question to get them talking (I have found that if you simply say, "Do you have any questions?" students will rarely ask, so be prepared with a question to ask them). Yesterday, a student brought up a question regarding Downward Dog and in explaining, I found that most students in class didn't understand the instruction to "lift your tailbone." This was a great opportunity to have a short anatomy discussion and to break down that pose further.

Anticipate what some of them may be experiencing and add instruction specific to it. As an experienced yoga teacher, you'll know the common challenges that newer students may face. Many may be feeling wrist sensitivity in Downward Dog, hamstring tightness in a forward fold, tight hips in Pigeon. Speak to these dynamics as you teach and offer suggestions to remedy the situation. Offer hands-on assists as well. Watch their bodies for signs they're uncomfortable; newer students will shake out their wrists; you'll see their thighs shaking in Downward Dog and you'll see their chest lift far away from their thighs in a forward fold. As always, teach to what you see; don't just offer these suggestions if no one in the room appear to be having the issue.

Help them with their props. New students won't understand what props to take and how to use them. In some classes, I begin with a quick explanation of how to use blocks, straps and blankets. If you're in a studio that has different block types, it's helpful to show them the difference. Also, if a student comes with a brand new mat that's curling up at the edges or a gym or other kind of exercise mat, get them a mat from the studio. Using the mat they came with will only be frustrating.

For the students that have trouble getting into Pigeon, help them prop their body up with blocks and a blanket. It will be hard for them to get into the pose, let alone manage their props as well.

Encourage them to come to any of your classes, even those that are not for Beginners. I often get the question, "Do you think I'm ready to take an All levels class?" from a beginning yoga student. I always encourage students to come to class, any class, and only suggest that they come with an open mind and a willingness to practice in a non-competitive, healthy fashion and to rest if they reach a point where they start to feel stressed. Your beginning students will look for your confirmation that they're ready but you want to encourage them and support the idea that they're ready now; they just need to bring a mindful attitude to class.

Acknowledge them for continuing to show up. When you start to see the same new faces from class to class, say something to acknowledge the student. " It's great to see you again. I can see you're developing a regular practice!" is a nice way to recognize them. This can be done in a professional and mindful way, so it's not to exclude anyone else or single one student out, but a friendly comment can let the student know that you notice the new healthy habit they're developing. For many students, it took a lot to show up once and now that they're in a new groove, it can be powerful for them if you notice.

Go to class a bit earlier than usual. If you're often running in five minutes before, take the time if possible, to go ahead of time. Make sure the studio and props are in tiptop order. Unless you work in a studio where there are assistants to manage this piece, be sure the studio is clean, props are stacked and ready to go and your mat (if you use one) is out. This will ensure that when you arrive, the room will be ready for your class.

If the props are far from the center of the room, take a few and put them near to your mat or center of the room. This will ensure that if you need one for a student, you don't have to climb over bodies and over to the corner to get what you need. Anticipate you'll need one because they'll forget—even though you'll mention it before class as something to pick up.

Help students find their way in the room. It can be intimidating for new students when they first walk in the studio. They are often self-conscious and put their mat down in the first available place just because they're nervous. Be there to help them find a place and if this is their first time, see if there's a spot in the middle or back of the room so they have some perspective and can see you clearly.

Acknowledge them before you dive into the flow. Especially in true beginner's classes, say a few words before class. It might just be a "Hello, my name is… How are you doing today?" It's not so much to get a response, which you most likely will not get, but more to ground you and them into the moment before jumping into the poses. If something inspires you to discuss, like a short overview of what you'll do, go ahead. But resist the urge to go into great detail as you'll just overwhelm them.

Once you start class, stay present. Speak to what is happening right in front of you, not to the routine in your head. This is a helpful tip for all of us, all the time, but even more so with beginners. It's easy to go on auto-pilot but you'll miss the most helpful thing to say, which might be as simple as reminding them to breathe.

Resist the urge to be "Rescuer". It's easy to want to be there to assist every student, fully. First of all, it's impossible. Second of all, recognize that part of the practice for them is to find their own way. Helping them tap into their own intuition by encouraging them to rest when they need to, modify when they need to, or breathe more when they feel challenged will be empowering for them. You're helping them realize that they can help themselves, even in unfamiliar territory.

Offer lots of modifications and Child's Pose. Know that students either won't know how to modify certain poses or won't do it out of fear they're doing "less than." Also know they won't rest unless you ask them to rest. This is another reason why it's great to really be present to what is in the room; you'll see they're tiring and you'll know it's a good time to rest.

If someone leaves, keep your eye on them but resist the urge to chase them. For some students, in that first experience, the best way they can care for themselves is to leave. If they stay in the lobby, try to put the class in Child's Pose, go out and encourage them back in. Ask them how they are feeling. Reserve judgment and don't make them feel badly. If they choose to leave, ask them to come back another time.

Leave time for ample rest. Those first few classes can be emotionally and physically exhausting. For many students, it took moving huge boulders of resistance to be there. Give them time to rest.

Invite them back to the studio. After closing the class, encourage them to come back to any class. Let them know when you will be back. Suggest that they resist the urge to over think their experience and keep an open mind and return as soon as possible. Let them know you are available after class for questions. Stay in the room. Stay friendly and relaxed. Know that if they do approach you, it most likely is with caution but welcome their questions.

Let's break down some of the components of a beginner's class in more detail:

The practice

When teaching beginners, we're trying to build a number of competencies:

- An awareness of the breath
- The technical ability to breathe in Ujjayi style
- Knowledge of the poses
- An understanding of the sequence
- A greater ability to listen to the body, rest when needed and push when appropriate
- An ability to appreciate stillness and connect to the meditative side of the practice

As a result, it's important that the poses we present and how we present them gives the students ample space to be able to experience all of these things. While we want to give beginners a balance between challenge and accessibility, it's helpful to remember that for pure beginners, the most essential yoga practice of 60-90 minutes will be challenge enough without ever doing an arm balance or anything outside the traditional postures.

As a result, sticking to a basic sequence is one of the first things to keep in mind when working with beginners. The actual postures in the sequence may vary from teacher to teacher, depending on background and training. My training by Baron Baptiste provided me with a solid sequence that is great for both beginners and more advanced students. It starts with Sun Salutations and moves through twists, balances, triangles, backbends, abdominals and hip openers. Whatever you select, use the first few Sun Salutations to explain the alignment for this section of the practice. Sun Salutations are done in just about every style of yoga and can be a complex sequence for a beginner to understand. Further, moving from High to Low Push Up can be wrought with errors in alignment and have potential ramifications for the stability of the shoulder joint. Demonstrate, assist, use essential language; all of these things are useful to beginners.

New students will not have an idea of how to use the breath in a yoga practice. Help them learn Ujjayi breathing by starting them seated on a block. Throughout class, cue them on breathing and remind them that holding the breath through difficult poses, while it might sound like a good idea, actually makes things harder. Help them see how inhaling can create length in the spine and breathing out in coordination with twisting can deepen twists. Help them learn to listen to their breath to get clues from their body as to how they're doing physically in the practice.

Remember that people learn differently; some will learn through your demonstration of a pose, while others will be fine listening to your verbal instruction. Some will respond best to hands-on assists and others will flinch when you try to assist them, unsure of what they're supposed to do during an assist. One of the things I love to do in beginner's classes is take a little time at the start to break down a posture. If you stick with this format each week, people can pick up on a few specific pointers and your class will take on a workshop feel. They'll feel like they're getting more than just a class and you'll develop a loyal group of followers.

This holds for all classes but especially in classes with beginners: stay present and watch them closely. Beginners in yoga may not have a good sense of how to gauge their energy levels and may push too hard, may not be breathing steadily or may be breathing too much. They can be overheating in heated classes and may be pushing to a point of complete exhaustion which is easier to do because there is much more energy expended when you're unsure how to do each pose. Be conscious of offering time to rest and give ample time at the end for at least 5 minutes of rest in shavasana.

The physical space

The physical space in which we practice yoga is part of an expression of the practice. If the space is messy, it creates a chaotic atmosphere and one in which it can be hard to focus. A clean space reflects care and respect and encourages others to show the same.

Beginners will be nervous and anxious when they arrive. Having a clean, organized space for them will encourage them to relax and settle down, while you're greeting students. Be sure props are available for them and that there are enough for each person. Sometimes people will grab more than one block and after 8 or 10 people arrive, if each takes two blocks, there might not be enough for everyone. Keep your eye on the blocks and if so, ask someone if they can give up one so everyone has at least one.

Mat placement can also be an issue with beginners. There's the issue of where to put it, how close to others, where to place props, how close to be to the wall and what direction to face. The more you can be available in the room to help them place their mats, the better. The other thing that can be helpful is to place mats for students that arrive close to starting time. There's nothing more anxiety producing for a new student than walking into a full yoga studio and having to look around and figure out where to put your mat. Or, worse than that, having to ask people to move their mats so there is space for your mat. Help the latecomers with mat placement by keeping an eye out for the open spots. Encourage the students already in the room to keep their mats on line and evenly spaced. This makes it much easier to fit in new students as they arrive.

One more thing about mats: If students arrive with brand new mats or mats that are not really yoga mats per se but more exercise mats (shorter and thicker), give them a rental mat. Don't worry about the rental fee in the moment; the idea is to get them on a mat that will support them in their practice. For brand new, slippery mats, one can usually get by with a small towel under the hands. For anyone with an exercise mat, they just need a new mat. You can catch them after class for the rental fee.

The use of props

When working with people unfamiliar with yoga, they won't know what props to take or how to use them, let alone where to place them so they're at the ready. Take some time at the beginning of class to let them know what props to use and where to place them. One of the classic signs of a beginner is that the blocks are at the back of the mat. This makes them hard to reach when you need them. Suggest before class that people move them to the front of the mat on the side.

Also take a few minutes to show them what each is used for at the beginning of class or in the first pose where you call out the use of a block, strap or blanket. In most sequences, the block will primarily be used as a prop and many people will not know where to place it or recognize that as you place it on different sides, it is flatter, longer or taller. Specifically suggest the use of a block in a pose, use it as a chance to demonstrate how to use it and speak to the alignment needed. In many poses, the block should be placed so the shoulder stacks over the wrist so that maximum leverage and stability is experienced. This isn't always intuitive for people so a quick demonstration will help.

For you, as the teacher, be sure you have quick access to props. You'll want to grab one for a student who forgot or you might need more than one block or a strap for someone and won't have time to run across to the prop area to retrieve one. Take a few out and place them in the center of the studio for easy access.

One more note about props: people can sometimes feel that using props is a reflection of their ability to practice yoga. They may be apprehensive about grabbing a block, especially if the person next to them isn't using one. Rather than saying, "If you'd like to use a block, place it under your right hand," simply say, "Place a block under the hand, stacking the shoulder over the wrist." In this way, you're stating it as a fact and if people chose for whatever reason not to use one, that's up to them. In this way, you're not making excuses for the beginners, or going into a long story about blocks not being for beginners; you're just saying, "use one."

The language used in teaching

My style and my training have always been focused on providing essential language. What does this mean? It means saying only what's needed and as clearly and succinctly as possible. This helps people hear you clearly, cuts down on confusion and preserves your energy (the more you say, the more energy you use to say it). For an in-depth review of what essential language for yoga teachers is like, see my chapter on the subject. In general, provide more information at the front end of each portion of the sequence and less on the second side. This means that you use the first part of the Sun Salutations to provide more instruction on alignment and less on the second. This allows people to start to integrate on their own and have space for quiet and hearing their breath. This works great with sides of the body; so, for instance, using the right side of the Triangle sequence to support students with alignment information and then on the second side, giving less instruction and more physical assisting (again, this is a great way for you to preserve your energy).

Assisting

As a teacher, you have many tools available to you in order to teach yoga and in order to build connection with the students in class. One wonderful way is assisting. Through assisting, you are able to acknowledge each student through hands-on touch and also give him or her reinforcement as to the alignment in the pose. There are also assists you can give that will deepen the experience of the pose by the student. While these should be used carefully, it is an option. Please refer to the chapter called, "Essential Assisting Tips" for an in-depth discussion of how to assist students effectively.

For purposes of our discussion here, there are a few key things to keep in mind when assisting:

- As a teacher, you need the confidence to include assisting in your teaching
- Assisting is touching another person and many times, it is a person

you don't know, or someone who has not specifically given you permission to touch them. As such, you must show confidence and clarity in your touch, as well as respect

- Be present as you assist, so to clearly communicate the action you desire to express
- Use assisting primarily as a tool to express proper alignment. Reinforce twisting, bringing joints in line or place blocks under hands in the right spot. These are all good examples of how to use assisting to communicate alignment.

There are many courses available that specifically teach assisting techniques. If your 200 HR teacher training did not include a section on assisting or you lack the confidence to integrate it in your teaching, invest in yourself and get the necessary training before adding assisting into your classes.

One note about building connection: Most students will love to get an assist but if you sense any hesitancy from the student or you feel that approaching the student would be detrimental, refrain. Also, it is up to you as a teacher if you wish to state at the beginning of class that you will be assisting. Some teachers like to state this, as a way to allow students to state that they do not wish to be assisting. In my experience, a student will rarely speak up in front of others to let you know that they are not interested in getting assisted. So, while you may wish to bring it up, be ready for someone to tell you while you are approaching them individually.

It goes without saying, but to be perfectly clear: Assisting is touching another person and should be approached with care and respect. Rather than looking at what is "wrong" with the pose that you can "correct" through your assisting, consider your assisting as another way to teach and to support the expression of the pose by the individual.

One last thing: If a student asks you to assist them in a particular pose (either just as you're teaching it or before class) remember that assisting is not a "by demand" technique. You not only need to be in good physical shape to effectively assist, but you need to be close to the student in order to do it. In large classes, this may or may not be possible when the particular requested pose comes up in the sequence. It is completely within your role as a teacher to let the person know that if it is possible, you will gladly provide it.

Closing Summary

One of the most important things to do with beginners is to be available. Come early and stay after class. Look for people who appear to be ready to ask a question but may be hesitant to approach you to ask. Smile and ask them how it's going. This may be the catalyst needed to strike up a conversation.

Also, remember as a teacher that working with beginners can be a dynamic process. There will be lots of extra movements, as people work to build stability in the poses. This is not uncommon in any class but with beginners, it may be more pronounced. Approach these classes with an easy-going, light attitude, rather than with one of rigidity and discipline. Keep a healthy perspective; you're helping people access a way to find greater health and the beauty of personal expression in each pose. There is no need to "get it right." Your role is to be there to help and support.

Chapter 20

Teaching Children's Yoga

Focus

Why teach yoga to children?

There has never been a more challenging time to be a child. Kids today live in a world that is full of distraction, unhealthy foods, academic demands and competition. Kids learn stress at a young age as they deal with negative images in the news or in their neighborhoods, broken families, increasing pressures to succeed in school, pressure to wear the "right clothes," be the "right weight" and have the coolest electronic device.

Schools are under increasing pressure to have their students perform more, with less. Budgets are being cut, while increased scrutiny is being placed on teachers and how they are managing their students.

One low cost tool that can be used to effectively strengthen both the body and mind of child is yoga. Yoga is a wonderful way for children to learn how to develop body awareness in a supportive, non-competitive environment. Yoga teaches children how to use their bodies in a healthy way and gives them stress management techniques through breathing, increased awareness, meditation and healthy movement.

Bringing yoga to children has amazing benefits. It provides them with tools and techniques for managing stress, increasing concentration, builds creativity, increases confidence as well as feeling part of the group. All these skills and behaviors have been demonstrated to improve their ability to learn and do well from an academic perspective. Yoga provided in the schools and other settings with children also provides the teachers with management techniques for the classroom instead of using punishment or isolation as way to deal with a challenging child. It allows them to also feel part of the learning process and gives them a regular activity they can integrate into their daily lesson planning.

Yoga can provide children with a way to develop a self-image that's strong and healthy and give them an alternative to succumbing to peer pressure, participating in non-productive activities and tuning out with constant attachment to the computer and television. Gandhi said, "Be the change you wish to see in this world" and at the core of that statement is the concept that one person can affect change by setting an example for others and by taking "right action." Kids who develop a strong self-image will become models for other kids and will be in a better position to grow into healthy adults.

Overall Considerations

Yoga is a wonderful way for children to learn how to develop body awareness in a supportive, non-competitive environment. Yoga teaches children how to use their bodies in a healthy way and gives them stress management techniques through breathing, increased awareness, meditation and healthy movement.

Yoga classes for children should provide elements from each of the foundations of a yoga practice (see below). As children increase in age, their level of awareness and capability increases along with their ability to sustain their attention for longer periods of time. As such, classes will contain the same elements but how they are pieced together will vary. Sessions with older children might have more vinyasa (flow sequencing) versus classes with younger children, which would bring these same elements to light through games and shorter vinyasa sequences.

Introducing yoga to children is an incredibly useful tool. It provides them with tools and techniques for managing stress, increasing concentration, builds creativity, increases confidence as well as feeling part of the group. All these skills and behaviors have been demonstrated to improve their ability to learn and do well from an academic perspective. Yoga provided in the schools or in other teaching settings (such as Boys and Girls Clubs) provides the teachers with management techniques for the classroom instead of using punishment or isolation as way to deal with a challenging child. It allows them to also feel part of the learning process and gives them a regular activity they can integrate into their daily lesson planning.

Foundations for all the Practices

Breathing: Yoga is called a breathing practice. Through deep breathing we learn a natural way to build connection as well as both energize and release tension and stress. Yoga breathing is a rhythmic process that improves blood flow, circulation and the delivery of fresh, oxygen rich blood to the brain. For young kids, breathing techniques are centered around short games and exercises meant to teach the different ways you can use breath to affect the way you feel in your body. As children grow older, more traditional yoga breathing techniques can be introduced. Children involved in athletics like soccer, running or other sports can use yoga breathing to increase their lung capacity. Breathing techniques can be used to increase focus, attention span and the ability to release tension in a healthy way.

Strengthening/Energizing: Newer students or those who have never tried yoga often are under the impression that while yoga builds flexibility it does not really increase strength. This is a true misunderstanding. Imagine having the strength to hold your body in the air while balancing on one arm or one leg? Imagine using isometric resistance to hold a position, like a squat or a standing posture while breathing deeply? Imagine developing the strength in your arms and legs and the flexibility in your spine to do five backbends in a row? These are all part of a vinyasa (flow) yoga practice and over time will build an intrinsic, fluid strength in your body. This is a very different kind of strength than one gets from lifting weights. It is built on a foundation of lengthening as well as strengthening the muscles. This provides strength as well as lightness in the body. While those with exceptional muscle strength can hold a yoga pose, the idea is to move the body with strength that comes from fluidity not one of holding and straining.

Children have different muscle composition depending on their age. In smaller children, their muscles are very flexible as well as their joints. The goal of yoga practice at this age is not so much on building strength but more around building an awareness of the intrinsic, internal quality of muscles. It also promotes muscle coordination as children learn the poses and how to connect one movement to the other. They build an awareness of their limbs in space. As children get older, yoga poses and sequencing is more traditional and can emphasize building strength through holding a pose for 3-5 breaths as well as introducing more challenging postures. Bodies that are strong from the inside out digest food better, maintain a healthy weight and can support the stress of carrying heavy loads, such as a backpack loaded with books. These bodies will also breathe better, work more efficiently and protect the more fragile joints of the body safely.

Balancing: Balancing poses are part of any traditional yoga practice and teach children that with increased focus to one point one can channel energy and increase attention in a natural way. Children who struggle with attention deficit disorder or who are easily distracted can improve their ability to focus by practicing balancing sequences. These poses also develop an intrinsic strength as kids learn to balance their weight on one leg, or an arm and a leg, while the body is positioned in a variety of ways. Balancing poses also evoke a more meditative feeling and while yoga is typically called "meditation in motion," balancing poses give kids a taste of stillness which is traditionally only found in a seated meditation. Stillness allows one to quiet the mind, which brings on a sense of natural peace. This becomes a wonderful technique in both kids and adults to deal with the stress of living in a chaotic world where constant stimulation is a regular part of life. It has been shown that constant stimulation is stressful to the body at a cellular level and raises the level of stress hormones. Living with constant stimulation and high levels of these stress hormones such as cortisol can damage the body. Bringing a daily dose of stillness can counter the effects of this and provide techniques to achieve stillness and calm despite living in our chaotic world.

Stretching/Lengthening: The opposite of strengthening is lengthening the body. With increased length comes increased flexibility. While having a strong body is great, a body that is only based on strength has no way to yield and bend. Muscles that only know strength can't move quickly and may actually pull on joints and bones as they shorten, as tight muscles tend to shorten. While we don't typically see this in young children, it's important to develop flexibility in muscles as well as building strength at an early age. A typical yoga practice with traditional postures stretches every muscle in the body and through intensive breathing and movement, muscles warm and become suppler. Supple, flexible muscles can give way when need be and support tender joints in a healthy, functional way. The typical analogy is the football player that needs not only strength, but also flexibility to allow him or her to move quickly and nimbly and be reactive to impact without fear of breaking a bone. Bodies built with yoga have the needed flexibility to be reactive to unforeseen impact and the physical demands of life.

Awareness/Focus: While certain parts of a yoga practice can be relaxing, the main goal of yoga is to create a greater sense of awareness and increase one's ability to focus. Some people have a misperception that through yoga's meditative qualities, one is almost lulled to sleep and the final yoga posture in class, Shavasana, mirrors sleep. Nothing could be further from the truth. Yoga is about creating awareness in the body and through the increased sense of connection to one's body, on a physical level, other avenues of consciousness open up as well. For many adults as well as children, the best place to start is with the breathing and with an increased focus on deep, rhythmic breathing.

Children have a wonderful awareness of their bodies, which can be cultivated through creative expression. Yoga provides kids with a wonderful way to not only express themselves but also start to build a strong connection between what they hear and integrating movements into the body. As we age, we lose our connection to our bodies, which we often see in a group yoga class as expressed in even a simple movement like raising your arms up above your head. It's not uncommon to see lots of variation when you ask an adult class to "reach to the sky." It comes from arms that are limited due to shoulder tightness to those with flexibility enough to raise the arms above the head but in a body that is totally disconnected.

Children that have awareness in their bodies and minds are more confident, stronger, have better posture, breathe better and have a sense of quiet strength. The ability to focus, like what we see in balancing postures, allows students to develop a sense of peace in the midst of chaos; and what better skill to teach our kids as they grow up in this ever-changing and increasingly chaotic world.

Flowing/Connecting/Integrating: The style of yoga that we will teach is called Vinyasa Power Yoga. While with small children we will teach this style of yoga more through the use of games versus a traditional practice, in all of the classes we will introduce the postures or asanas and will focus on connecting the postures together through connecting movements. The word "vinyasa" means "flow" and in this context, "flow" means the removal of blocks or decreasing resistance. Through rhythmic breathing, interconnecting movements and the postures, we will start to give the body a taste of what it means to have liquid movement, like water flowing out of a faucet. The other quality that this builds in children of all ages is awareness that all our movements are a series of coordinated efforts between muscles, bones, joints and nerves. As children get older, they are more able to isolate different muscle groups in a posture and get more sophisticated about movements; things like keeping the arms lifted in Warrior 1, while at the same time, dropping the shoulders to relax them.

All these things together increase a child's sense feeling integrated. This is a sense that we are not only ourselves a connected unit comprised of many different parts, but we live in a world where we can do things individually but we are connected to each other as well as nature and all the things around us. This builds a sense of feeling connected to others and can combat feelings of isolation, feeling "different" from others, and loneliness.

Meditation/Relaxing/ Slowing down/Centering: One of the most commonly recognized qualities of a yoga practice is its meditative nature. Through stillness, whether that's holding a balancing posture or sitting in meditation or even through the traditional flowing series of a vigorous vinyasa sequence, there is a calming, soothing quality. Athletes talk about being in "the zone" while traditional yoga theory refers to it as "pratayhara;" a sense of turning inward, bringing the focus to one thing and losing a sense of time.

While small children won't get a full sense of this in their classes, as they're more filled with games and full body movements, there are portions of even the youngest kids classes that are centered on stillness and turning inside. In classes of kids that are in the 4-6-age range, they may only be able to be in stillness for 1-2 minutes. But as children grow, their ability to sustain meditation in a more traditional seated position or lying down increases. And they are also able to develop a taste of the "zone" feeling discussed earlier. For young children, it is helpful to give them something to do as they as lying on the floor. It is also helpful to place them in relationship to each other to make a "game" out of it. Have them lie in a circle, feet touching in the center. Ask them to lie down and close their eyes and think of a "favorite color" or a "favorite place to visit" or "favorite toy." Ask them to keep the thought to themselves. See if they can rest for a few minutes and then have them come up to seated and share what came to mind.

As children get older they can tolerate rest with less talking from you as the teacher, but it is an ideal time to help them to pull together their experiences on the mat to how it can be used off the mat as well.

Suggested supplies for teaching children's yoga

The list below is a suggested list only and can be used as a starter kit for a teacher beginning to teach children's yoga. While many of these items are primarily used when teaching younger children, even as children approach the teen years and well into their teens, they can learn from being creative with props such as the items below. Use of these items will be outlined in further sections of this manual.

Straws
Balloons
Beanbags
Crayons
Construction paper
Pinwheels
Blowing bubbles
Long rope
Large exercise ball
Pipe cleaners
Beads and string
Flashcards with animal pictures
Books that show the muscles and bones of the body
Stickers
Name tags
Yoga Pretzel Card Deck (found on Amazon)
My Daddy is A Pretzel (found on Amazon)
Any commercially made flashcards that have pictures of animals
Big Picture books

Yoga Activities by Age Group

Toddler to 3 years old

Breathing:
- Yoga cards with breathing exercises
- Holding the breath and counting
- Placing hands on the belly and feeling breath as it moves in and outBreathing as different animals: Bee, Snake, Dragon
- Blowing bubbles
- Using pinwheels
- Blowing cotton balls with straws

Strengthening/Energizing:
- Game: Yogi Says (based on the classic Simon Says game)
- Game: Pretend to be an animal
- Game: Yoga Journey
- Song: "If You're Happy and You know it"
- Game: Show me a way to stretch your body
- Flashcards with animal pictures

Balancing:
- Make a circle- tree pose, airplane
- Balance beanbag on head- tree pose, airplane
- Walk the tightrope
- Stretching/Lengthening
- Touch the sky
- Touch your toes
- Animal poses
- Pose cards

Awareness/Focus:
- Balancing and focusing on one spot
- Breathing and feeling the belly
- Breathing and noticing and naming how you feel
- Flowing/Connecting/Integrating
- Songs
- Do 2 or 3 poses in a row, repeat 3 times

Meditating/Relaxing/Slowing down/Centering:
- "Show me what relaxed looks like"
- Bring feet to center of circle. Lie down and think of (Favorite color, favorite place, favorite animal) Come up and tell us what came into your mind

Specific considerations for this age group:

- Come with a plan but don't expect to use it!
- Have a few "go to" games to use when children are struggling to focus
- Use positive language instead of "please don't do that"
- "Tell" what we will do rather than "ask" or give choices but no more than two
- Singing is a great way to capture the attention of children
- Use stickers as rewards for job well done
- Let children be where they are, even if they are not participating. Re-direct as needed for disruptive children but allow individual kids to watch if that is all they can handle
- Have special "jobs" for children that are disruptive to the group (holding a book, turning the page, watching the clock, etc)

4-8 years old
Breathing:
- Holding breath for different counts
- Back to back breathing
- Feeling breath
- For older children, talking about lungs and oxygen
- For older children, talking about different kinds of breath and how it connects to feeling different things (stressed, excited, happy)

Strengthening/Energizing:
- Pose cards
- Basic standing poses
- "Be the teacher"
- Balancing:
- Tree pose individually and together
- Bean bag on head and walk across room
- Tightrope walk, forward, backward, on one leg

Stretching/Lengthening:
- Dog dog/Peeing dog
- While in poses, ask children "what am I stretching?" and help them identify body parts
- Pipe cleaners and discussion about spine
- Bending over exercise ball
- "Show us your favorite yoga pose"
- Awareness/Focus:
- Drawing

Flowing/Connecting/Integrating:

- Short sequences of standing poses
- Yoga journey: Have children participate in suggesting what comes next in the story
- Kids in a circle; do first child's pose, then next child's pose, then first and second, then third and so on.
- Lay cards on the floor of poses and put them together in a sequence

Meditating/Relaxing/Slowing down/Centering:
- Resting and thinking of fun places to visit, favorite animals, favorite colors
- Body parts as heavy as working through shavasana
- Squeeze/ release different body parts
- Specific considerations for this age group:
- Greater levels of participation
- Greater levels of verbalization
- Greater levels of focus and following direction
- Increased resistance to following directions
- Use stickers as rewards

Pre/Teen and Teen years (elementary and high school)

Breathing:
- Teaching breathing with movement
- Discuss oxygen, it's role in exercise, the affect of rhythmic breathing on lung capacity. Help children see how yoga will improve sports performance by increasing lung capacity

Strengthening/Energizing:
- Traditional vinyasa
- Holding poses and asking children "what muscles am I working?"

Balancing:
- Traditional poses
- Partner balancing poses which emphasize teamwork

Stretching/Lengthening:
- Traditional poses
- Pipe cleaners as spine, discussion of backbends, backbends over the ball and on floor

Awareness/Focus:
- Ask kids how yoga feels in their bodies
- Use books on anatomy to help kids identify body parts
- Ask kids for feedback about how they feel in different poses ("was this easy or challenging?")
- Have kids write on flashcards how they feel when they practice

yoga to help them identify sensations and feelings

Flowing/Connecting/Integrating:
- Link poses together after showing separately

Meditating/Relaxing/Slowing down/Centering
- Shavasana
- Closing eyes and using visualization

Specific considerations for this age group:
- Help kids see how yoga translates "off the mat"
- Help kids to identify how they feel with words
- Ask kids what they think of when they hear the word "yoga"
- Use partner poses to help kids work together and challenge themselves

College years

Breathing: Teaching Ujjayi (as tolerated)

Strengthening/Energizing: Traditional sequencing

Balancing: Traditional poses

Stretching/Lengthening

Awareness/Focus:
- Talk to students about the value of staying in a pose and focusing on one spot
- Encourage students to provide feedback about how it felt to focus on one spot

Flowing/Connecting/Integrating:
- Share what 'vinyasa' means
- Kids at this age can follow a more traditional vinyasa but keep instruction essential as they are frequently overwhelmed and still distractible

Meditating/Relaxing/Slowing down/Centering:
- Shavasana
- Use visualization exercises that they can relate to (being in a warm place, going on vacation, see yourself relaxed and focused)

Specific considerations for this age group:
- Physically capable of more traditional vinyasa flow
- Modifications may be needed depending on physical condition of students
- Challenges to focus
- Help students understand applicability of yoga to their lifestyle

General Yoga Inspired Games
- Om/Namaste: Based on Red/ Light Green light, teaches kids the meaning of both Sanskrit words and allows kids to do different movements to go to the person who's 'it.'
- Put children in a circle and each child gets to pick something to help 'warm up' the body. Explain what 'warming up' means
- Obstacle course
- Yoga kick ball
- What is favorite yoga pose?
- "Be the yoga teacher"
- Balancing game: Partner up and have one child balance a beanbag on the top of the other child's head while that child holds balance
- Back bending limbo to music
- Down Dog Train with snakes crawling underneath
- Bringing stories to life
- Partner poses

Considerations for the teacher
- Be ready at all times to be expressive, creative and outgoing
- Managing children that refuse to participate or are disruptive to the group
- Managing children that pick on other kids
- Running, hitting other kids, using silly language
- Working with kids in the same class in different age groups
- Managing your frustration
- Being prepared
- Staying positive
- Being a role model
- Helping children use language that reinforces their capabilities
- Setting guidelines for participation
- Everything you do and say has the potential to be absorbed, even if in the moment, it seems as if the children are not paying attention

Things to avoid when teaching children
- Negative language
- Threatening ("If you don't stay on the mat, I'm going to tell your mother")
- Headstands
- Pulling on arms or legs or head

Closing Summary

Yoga is a rewarding and inspirational practice to teach to people of all ages and with children, there is a special fondness you can develop if you show up with a plan and with no expectations. While teaching yoga for children requires an abundance of energy and creativity as well as an ability to think of one's feet, it can provide teachers with a renewed sense of inspiration as they approach teaching their more traditional adult classes. Teaching to kids is fun, energetic and can give us, as adults, a way to stay connected to the most essential qualities for yoga: an open heart, an open mind and presence.

Sample Lesson Plans

4 years old (and up to teen years) Class

- Warm up game: " Hello my name is X and I like to
  _____ " Have children describe what they like to do
  to warm up the body. Explain what it means to "warm up."

- Balancing Game: Balancing game: Partner up and have one child
  balance a beanbag on the top of the other child's head while that
  child holds balance. Add balancing poses after the game

- " Two Yogi's were walking thru the forest and they saw a
  _____ ": Hand out the Pretzel cards to the kids, one to each kid.
  Lead off with the beginning of a story, " There were two yogis walking thru the forest. They met a ____ " and start with one child. See
  what pretzel card they have, have them read it to the group (or you
  read it) and then we all do the pose. Then continue w/ the story till
  you get thru all the kids and their cards. Try to pick cards that make
  sense (cobra, dog, river, etc)

- Spine Discussion: Discuss spine, have them point to their spine, on
  mom or dad have them touch spine. Show them different ways to
  bend spine. Then do backbending on ball and limbo stick, to music.

- Shavasana

Teen Yoga Class

- What is Yoga? Discuss quickly
- What do we need to give our bodies in order to do yoga? Breath,
  oxygen
      Bring Balloons and have them fill up balloons
      Talk about how balloons are like lungs
      Show them where on the body the lungs are
      Discuss how the more we fill them, the more oxygen they dis-
  tribute
      Do breathing exercises with them on their backs with hands on
  bellies- do different breathing exercises on backs
- Yoga has POSES called ASANAS (have them say it). Tell them

about Sanskrit and India- the history of yoga- a little bit.

- Discuss how yoga poses work in the WHOLE BODY but different poses help us get better at certain things and help us feel certain things:
- Poses to help us feel strong: (write on white board)
- Warrior 1
- Warrior 2
- Thunderbolt
- Triangle
- Down Dog
- Plank
- Poses to help us feel balanced:
- Tree
- Dancers
- Side plank
- Mountain (with eyes closed)
- Navasana
- Poses to help us rinse out stress:
- Prayer twist
- Knee down twisting crescent
- Poses to help us open our heart:
- Up dog
- Bridge
- Wheel

- Do a vinyasa
- Partner poses-put kids w/their bigs and pick two partner poses they can do (bring cards)

- Shavasana
- Closing activity: Have them write down on the card and on the master board:

YOGA HELPS ME TO FEEL:_____

Mixed Age/ Family Yoga Class

<u>Start out with Yogi Says</u>

Be the yogi first and do a few poses and stretches

TRY TO TRICK THEM, especially the little kids
Then, turn it over to the participants, especially the kids, to see if they want to be the yogi and give us suggestions about what stretches or poses to do
Can crown some of the little kids as they come up and "be the yogi", if the group size works for that (use party crown)

Breathing Exercises

Some basic standing stretches with deep breathing in and out
Ask them why breathing is so important in yoga
While standing, have them place hands on their bodies to feel their sides expand with every breath
Have them do Lion's breath. If little ones present, have them do it on their hands and knees

Balancing

Walk magic tightrope (rope)
Then, balancing poses
Tree
Eagle
Dancers
Airplane

Backbending

Limbo stick- to music
Bridge
Wheel

Partner Poses

Large group:
Forest of trees
Sky divers
Adults in Down dog, kids run thru
Adults make mountaintop, kids run thru

Partner poses:

Dancers facing each other
Boat with feet touching each other
Back to back sitting and up to seated standing position
Down dog on down dog
Back to back child's pose

<u>Yoga Journey (if the class is older kids and parents, do a traditional vinyasa)</u>

We're going on a yoga journey where we'll meet lots of different animals and people and things in nature

First, we'll stand tall like a mountain
Then we'll stretch our arms out like the sun (triangle)
We'll fly like an eagle
And soar like an airplane
Then, we'll run into a silent, strong warrior, with arms reaching high to the sky
We'll be strong with roots like a tree
And be light on our feet like a dancer

To floor

We'll meow like a cat
Roar like a lion
Bark like a dog
Pee like a peeing dog
Roar like a lion
We'll slither thru the grass like a cobra
And then be still like a rock (child's pose)
We'll sail like a boat
And
Make like a river (seated forward bend)
We'll float like a butterfly (badda konasana with arms like wings)
And bring our hands to our heart center and say

PEACE!

Chapter 21

Teaching Private Yoga Sessions

Focus

Working with people one on one is a great way to teach yoga. In your time as a teacher, private yoga sessions may become a large part of what you offer. There are many benefits to teaching privately. It is a great way to learn how to customize the sequence to meet the individual needs of the person. Also, because of the one on one attention, the rate you charge is most likely more than the rate you are paid for teaching a studio class. That aspect aside though, teaching privates is a great way to hone your skills as a teacher and deepen your relationship to yoga practice and with your students.

Overall Considerations

Considerations as a Student

Sometimes, students are not sure if a private would be appropriate for them. In my experience, there are many good reasons to take a private. As a yoga teacher, it's a good idea to have these reasons in mind, so you can share them with people as they ask why they might invest in a private session. They include:

Students will learn proper alignment. Everyone learns differently. Some people are more visual, while others are more auditory. In a private lesson, students will learn in a way that suits the way their brain works. As a teacher, you'll learn this as well in terms of what works best with the individual. Learning proper alignment is key to working efficiently on the mat and also building strength and flexibility without getting hurt.

Students will learn how to breathe in a way that is particular to yoga practice, called Ujjayi breathing. In yoga, breathing is the key to fueling the muscles as well as generating that sense of overall calm that comes with practice. It comes from stimulating the relaxation response in the nervous system. However, it won't happen if students are unsure how to breathe in this Ujjayi style of breathing. In an individual session, you have a chance to really show someone how to do this and get their feedback as to how it feels. There are other styles of breathing as well and you can work these in too.

Students will learn how to modify poses in a way that is unique to their body. As we learn yoga, our body can be better supported if certain modifications are done. These modifications may or may not involve using props, but either way, they are critical to helping build the pose properly and safely without doing too much too soon. A yoga teacher can help a student learn how to modify. This also comes in handy if a student gets injured in a particular way and wants to still practice.

Students will learn how to use props. All yoga studios have props and people sometimes are not sure how to use blocks, straps or blankets. In a private session, students will have the time to explore how to use this equipment to enhance their practice.

Students will learn how to work with any injuries or conditions they might have, that in the past, might have made someone hesitant to attend a group class. Sometimes people come to a private session because they are injured or working with a physical challenge that is either temporary or permanent. A private yoga teacher can help a student set up a sequence and use props in a way that allows for safe practice.

Students can explore meditation as an additional wellness tool. Sometimes people come to yoga with an interest in developing a meditation practice as well. In a private session, students can learn about different styles of meditation and practice yoga together. A short, seated meditation after a 45-minute yoga session can be a wonderful experience and one that leaves a healthy imprint on the body and mind.

Students can learn challenging poses with one-on-one support. If students want to learn arm balances or other challenging poses, working with someone privately can be an approach. It can give them the support they need as well as that initial boost of confidence that comes once you get into that pose for the first time. We will explore this more in depth later as we discuss the different kinds of students that may invest in private sessions.

Students can do yoga privately rather than with others and can schedule the session at their convenience. Sometimes people come to private sessions simply because they prefer practicing alone and they can't get to the studio when classes are held. They also may appreciate the one on one, hands-on instruction versus being part of a crowded class.

Students can ask questions as you teach. Sometimes, in my group classes, a person will spontaneously ask a question. I know it can break people from their concentration but I'm sure there are lots of other questions that are left unsaid. In a private session, students can ask questions on the spot as they are in a pose. It's a very effective way to learn.

Students will receive physical assists during the session in addition to learning the poses. When students receive a private lesson, you will be giving hands-on assists while they are in the poses. Assisting is another way for a teacher to communicate how to do the poses from an alignment perspective.

Considerations for you as teacher

While teaching yoga to a group or an individual may involve similar sequences and poses, the techniques you use may be a bit different and there are certainly unique practical considerations as well. Let's consider some of what you'd need to think about as a teacher before you host your first private session.

Decide where you will provide private lessons. Some studios will let you rent space for a small fee. If you have a space in your home, make sure it's free of clutter, is clean and you have enough space for both the student and yourself, as you move around them on the mat.

Pets are great but have them off on their own during your session. I have a dog and she loves when people come to practice at the house. Once she greets the student, I have her in the bedroom and put up a pet gate so she can see us but isn't underfoot. Be aware when first time students visit that not everyone is dog or cat friendly. If you notice any wariness on the part of the person as they first arrive, bring your pet right away into the other room. I also am very careful to avoid them stepping on the student's mat while we're setting up.

Invest in quality mats and props. Even though most students will come prepared with a mat, they most likely will not have a block, blanket or strap. Spend a little money and invest in a few good mats, 2 blankets (great for under hips in Pigeon), two cork blocks (more stable than foam) and two straps. Be sure these mats stay clean and are only used for private sessions (don't use them yourself).

Ask questions before the session to understand the student's goals. If you make the appointment with the student in person, get an understanding of what they'd like to learn. You'll discuss more once they arrive for their first session but it's always helpful to get a general idea before they arrive. If you make the appointment over the phone or email, ask via that method.

Once the session is set up (via email or phone), confirm with the student 24 hours in advance. This helps to ensure their arrival, as sometimes, students forget. Have their phone and email and confirm via email. Let them know that if they're unable to attend, it's helpful to have at least 24 hours notice. While this is not like a doctor's appointment, you want the student to respect not only your time but their own. Also, as you get busier as a teacher, you may have other students you can fit into the time slot if someone cancels.

When the student arrives for the first session, have a seat and help them feel comfortable. You'll be the one to set the tone at this first session. Most students will be nervous, especially if they're in your home. It will be unfamiliar to them and they'll most likely feel self-conscious. Sit down, ask some open-ended questions: "I know we talked on the phone already. Let's talk a bit more about what you'd like to work on." Let them set the pace in this first session. I once had a woman come and we talked about her personal struggles with weight loss for the first 20 minutes. For many students, you are acting as a health coach as well as yoga teacher.

If your student has a specific injury they're working with or a medical condition, do some research before they arrive. Be prepared with ideas for a sequence but keep an open mind. Start with some seated breathing to get the student connected to their breath. Move on from there to stable poses, such as Cat/Cow or lying on the floor and pressing into Upward Dog or Cobra. You'll be doing diagnosing as you go in this first session, so keep an open mind. Your experience and ability to be creative as a teacher will be critical here.

Be generous with assisting. Many students love private sessions because they get lots of assists in yoga poses. It's like a massage and a yoga practice rolled into one! Be sure you feel comfortable around assisting. If not, ask a friend if you can practice on them a few times (you'll have friends lining up for this!).

Set your rate. This of course, happens before you offer the service. Generally speaking, teachers charge anywhere between $80-$125 for a private session for a one hour meeting but you may want to set a different rate depending on the circumstances (where it is, if travel is involved, etc). Let the student know the rate beforehand and the methods of payment you accept. If you'd like to accept credit cards, check out www.squareup.com.

Make sure you have liability insurance and create a waiver for signature at the first session. All yoga teachers should carry liability insurance. Check out www.phly.com for coverage. Also, have the student sign your release form when they first arrive. If you're looking for a sample form, I"ve included one at the back of the book.

Always be safe. If a student asks you to come to their home for a session, be sure you feel safe around the circumstances. If you prefer to hold sessions only in a public place, such as a studio, let the student know. If you're willing to travel to their location, make sure you ask in advance what space will be provided and be sure you include in your rate a payment factor to compensate for your travel time and the convenience to the student.

General themes for teaching private sessions

Given that people come to private yoga sessions for different reasons, you have an opportunity as a teacher to create some custom sequences for students to help them experience the practice safely and with integrity. Let's review some general themes, inspired by the list of reasons students would book a private session, and discuss the kinds of things you might do.

The Beginner: These students are great to work with because they are eager and open. The fact that they have set up a private yoga session with you shows great motivation to learn and build a solid foundation. It's also a great opportunity for you to show them correct alignment before they start to build unhealthy habits in practice.

Begin your session with a focus on the breath and how to create Ujjayi breathing. Move into teaching Sun Salutation A and B, as these two sequences will cover many things, including the alignment in Downward Dog, Upward Dog and Warrior 1; moving from High to Low Push Up and synchronizing breath to movement.

In a one-hour session, the above offering may take at least 30 minutes. Use the remaining time to cover one balancing pose, such as Tree, to allow the student to feel grounded and experience the benefits of balancing poses. Move on to the floor to present one or two poses on the belly, such as Locust and Bow and then move onto the back. Include a Bridge pose and then finish with Pigeon and Shavasana.

The above-suggested sequence will give your student an overall experience that covers the whole body. Go at a pace that meets the student's need and enter into the session with no agenda. Your role is to start with an intention but stay open to the questions the student has and allow ample time for adjustments and to explore each one.

I like to end each session with a few minutes for questions and then ask the student if he or she would like to set up a subsequent session. If not on the spot, I leave it open for the person to contact me whenever they wish.

The Injured Student: Students may come to you when they are returning to yoga after resolving an injury or while they are experiencing an injury and they wish to see if it's possible to continue their practice. While there is no way in this chapter to review every single possible injury, there are some things you can keep in mind when working with students in these two categories.

The first thing to ask the student is if their physician has cleared them to do yoga or related activities. If they have not, then you should suggest they do so before meeting with you for the first time (ideally, this will come up when they are trying to set up an initial session with you). Certainly anyone that is in physical therapy or someone who is post-surgery should have the blessing of a physician before starting a yoga practice.

Upon meeting the student, the first thing to understand is the nature of their injury or what injury has since resolved. Remember that it's important to not only know specifically what it is or was, like a herniated disc or Achilles tendonitis (although this is important too), but to understand how it impacted them. It's one thing to know the traditional clinical presentation of a particular injury, but this does not take into account the presentation in the individual. The severity of the injury, the nature of the person's body before the injury and their healing ability as well as the treatment they received or are still receiving all will have an impact on how that particular injury presents.

I like to ask questions about their current pain level, if pain wakes them at night (always a telling indicator), if the pain shows up during the day while they are doing their activities of daily living, such as driving, picking up groceries or sitting. Using the answers to these questions, I start to compile a mental note of movements that we may want to avoid all together (such as forward bending) or movements we need to approach with caution.

Once you have a general idea of the kind of injury, the nature of the injury, how it presents in the student and what movements to avoid, you can begin to present poses and see how he or she does. Allow lots of time and use props to support the person. As I said above, it's outside the scope of our work here to review every single kind of injury and present a modified practice but it is safe to say that starting with a seated pose and introducing deep breathing is always a great place to start. This can even be done in a chair for someone for whom sitting on the floor or a block is impossible.

Ask questions as you're moving through the sequence to see how the person is feeling. Remember that people will not always say if they are experiencing pain because they may be embarrassed or may be trying to appear strong. When you have 10 minutes left in the session, allow a full five minutes for Shavasana, being sure to support the person with props. Take the last five minutes of the session to ask what worked, what didn't and see how the student feels, both mentally and physically.

The Older Student: This is a bit of a tricky category because who is to say what age constitutes an "older" student? Certainly there is much more of a grey area here when we try to categorize someone as "older" but generally speaking, we can say this refers to people over 55 years old. Now, having said that and especially if you are a reader that is over 55 years of age and in excellent shape, you may be saying, "Hey, I don't need a modified yoga practice because of my age!" To you I say, "Awesome!" But, in my experience, what I find in my teaching is that there are many people in this age group who have never tried yoga and are interested, but due to lack of physical activity, are de-conditioned. So, perhaps the better name for this category is "Older and Deconditioned Students."

In working with someone like this, it's similar to working with a beginner. You'll want to start with the breath, as a way for the student to build connection to the body and to start to relax. Begin to work through a basic sequence and notice how the person is doing. Ask for feedback. One thing that can come up is the person may have a hard time moving from the floor to standing, as in Sun Salutations A and B. If that is the case, switch to presenting standing poses first and then move to the floor.

Remember to present all modifications, such as dropping the knee in Crescent Lunge, using a wide stance in Warrior 1, using blocks under the hands in Upward Dog or doing alternates such as Cobra instead. Work at a steady pace but allow time for the student to breathe and experience the pose. Watch for signs of stress, such as panting, redness in the face and shaking through the legs. Be generous with your offering of Child's Pose but be focused also on presenting a steady flow. These students (or anyone for that matter) should not be "babied" but should have adjustments made to the standard practice to accommodate them as they are gaining strength.

The Advanced Student: By "advanced," I'm referring to a student who has been practicing for a few years and is coming to you to learn specific poses or to learn new ways to find challenge in the practice. Sometimes students are looking also to correct bad habits or they could be coming merely because they enjoy the one-on-one time they get in a private session.

If they are there to learn some specific poses, it's helpful if you as a teacher can do them, so check with the student when they set up the session on what poses they'd like to learn. If you do run into a request that you cannot do, explain to the person that the pose in question is not part of your particular practice and look for an alternative or be open to the idea of teaching the pose from an "alignment only" perspective.

If the student is looking for a correction or confirmation that they are "doing it right" (this comes up a great deal), approach the first session as you would with a beginner, understanding that the student will be able to approach each pose with greater ease than a beginner but you should look for all the same general things you'd look for when working with a beginner.

If the student is coming to you more for the connection and attention one gets through a private session, look for ways to present challenge. This may not be only through the poses presented but could be through pace, sequence presented, moving deeper into some of the more traditional poses or having each session focus on a theme, such as inversions or twists.

The Corporate Executive Student: This is a bit of a tricky classification. This refers to the working corporate executive that may be seeing you because a friend referred them, or perhaps they've had health concerns and want to take better care of their physical and mental health. These are all great reasons and certainly something for you to build on together. However, in my experience, these students can be highly distractible, may have little to no yoga experience and may be self-conscious and nervous. Now, these qualities can apply to anyone and that's why I'm hesitant to classify them as qualities of this type of student. However, despite that, they can appear in students with this background so we will progress in our exploration here.

These students, given their work-a-holic lifestyle may also have a hard time putting their phone off to the side and on silent while you practice. Encourage them to leave their phone in the other room while you teach and if necessary, leave the ringer on, but at least in this case, they won't be checking email during your session. I also find that this kind of student, given their long work hours and extended computer use, will have very tight shoulders and hips. I also have a student who literally has shifted the position of his head forward over his chest so we work in each session to re-align his head on top of his spine.

For these students, the approach can be very much like the beginner; use the basics of breathing, alignment and the essential poses to build a connection to the body. For these students, just the mere work to breathe, be away from technology and be taking action to do something healthy can be very powerful. Give them ample time at the end to rest and be open to questions at the end. Look to integrate poses to help them open tight hips and shoulders and leave them with a few poses they can do at the office to stretch these tight parts.

Closing Summary

Working with people one-on-one is a great way to build a deeper bond with a student and be "of service" to someone looking to learn, deepen or modify their practice. It's a great way for you as a teacher to apply your knowledge in a comprehensive way, pulling together all that you know and applying it to an individual situation. Also, because the student will ask questions along the way, it's a great way to test your own knowledge of yoga and it's applicability in different people.

Remember to stay open, drop your defenses and stay focused on being of service. If something comes up that you do not know, let the student know you will research it and get back to them. Look for helpful, credible ways to stay in touch with your private students, including sending articles and videos that highlight things of specific use to them and being responsive to scheduling future sessions.

Chapter 22

Finding, Booking and Teaching Corporate Classes

Focus

One of the wonderful things about yoga's growth is that it's now offered outside the traditional setting of a studio and has made its way into offices and private settings, like training centers and schools. This has expanded the opportunities for yoga teachers so they can now pursue private teaching. Private gigs give teachers a chance to be the "expert" in a setting where typically no other yoga classes are offered and also gives them more leeway in setting a rate for classes (when compared to negotiating a rate with a studio owner).

Corporate yoga is seen by employers as a way to contribute to employees' overall health. It's also a great way to help employees work better both individually and in teams and can improve their perceptions of their employer. As yoga classes can be a low cost investment when compared to other wellness initiatives, it's no surprise that many employers are jumping on the yoga bandwagon.

Finding these teaching opportunities, booking them and teaching the classes requires a slightly different approach to finding, booking and teaching studio classes. We'll review considerations for each of these components below.

Overall Considerations

Finding Corporate Yoga Classes

Just as we discussed before, networking is the best way to find a teaching job. While some websites may post leads, it's still the best way. Here are some other ways to find a corporate teaching opportunity:

Ask your friends where they work: Ask your friends where they work and if they have ever had onsite yoga classes. Get a sense from them about the company culture. Many start-ups for instance, have a corporate culture that supports onsite wellness programs, especially because employees work around the clock. See who you know that can lead you to a possible gig.

Look for listings of the "Best Places to Work" in your city: I live in Boston and each year, the Boston Globe puts out a list of the "Top Employers" in the city, along with the Boston Business Journal. These lists note employers who have created a supportive and fun work environment and provide tangible benefits to their employees. Many have onsite wellness programs. Find these employers and cold call them or better yet, find someone you know who works there.

Call your old employers: Many yoga teachers left corporate gigs to teach yoga full-time. Now is the time to go back to your old employer as a free agent yoga teacher and see if you can get back in to teach classes.

Look for stories in the popular media that mention onsite employer wellness programs and pitch to those companies: There are stories all the time on the internet and television highlighting companies that are being creative in keeping their employees active. Set up a Google alert for "News about Employee Wellness" and see what you get. These are employers that are ripe for your pitch regarding onsite classes.

Booking Corporate Yoga Classes

Know your rate: Before you go into any negotiation about a corporate yoga (or any other kind of) yoga opportunity, you must know your hourly rate. This is critical for any business and it is a combination of your experience, value and your cost of doing business. You must know what you need to do the job and you must know the lowest rate you can accept and still make things work for you. Don't forget to take into account travel time as well. The longer you travel, the more that teaching gig will impact your ability to take on another class that same day. There is a cost to you for one gig taking up a significant chunk of your time during the day.

Define the length of time for the series: Corporate yoga programs should have a start and end date. While a client may renew after the end of the first series of 6-8 classes, setting it up as a series allows for both parties to evaluate the program before renewing. This can be helpful if either party wants to renegotiate the terms. This can be very helpful for the teacher, who, after teaching the first series, may find that there are aspects of the program that need to be modified.

Determine who will pay for the classes: Corporate yoga classes can be a paid for fully by the employer, fully by the employees or can involve some kind of cost sharing arrangement where the employer pays part and the employees pay a per class fee. Some arrangements may involve employees pre-paying for the series of classes (another good reason to offer classes in a series). How you chose to go will be a function of the employer's needs, the company culture, the nature of the relationship between the employer and employees, as well as a sign of how much the employer values offering the classes to employees.

Also, don't forget to include your requirements. If you're teaching full-time, you may be very dependent on a regular teaching rate per class. If the employer is unwilling to pay you a set rate per class and instead wants to leave it to the employees to pay as the classes are held, this will result in a variable rate to you. If your budget can't handle this variability, you may not be able to agree to that option.

Note: Don't be afraid to walk away from a teaching opportunity if the conditions are not right for you. If the client is only willing to set up a pay schedule based on their needs or are asking you to drop your rates in order to get the job, be wary of moving forward. Don't feel as if you need to justify your rate but do be sure, before you share your rate, to share information about you, your training, recommendations and other things that will demonstrate your experience.

One more thing: if the potential client is only interested in discussing your rate, and in the first contact with you, asks what is your rate, also be wary and resist the urge to simply share your standard rate. There are many variables to consider with corporate jobs, which may all impact your rate (travel, length of class, equipment needed, etc). Always steer the potential client to a discussion about their needs first and finding out what they want before you go into a discussion about rate.

Decide on the details regarding mats, props and room location

before the first class: Take the time to see the location where you'll be holding class. Decide if there is any room set up to be done each week and if so, who will be responsible for clearing the room. Find out if you need to bring mats or props and if so, be sure to think through how you will transport both as these can be quite heavy to carry.

Write out an agreement that clearly spells out the terms of the program: I have a standard Statement of Work that outlines the details of any teaching opportunity (non-studio) that I negotiate. This helps both myself and the client see in writing exactly what we have agreed to, which has usually been discussed both in person and via several emails. This document pulls all the details together and requires the signature of both parties. While it mentions contact and program information, one of the most important sections is on payment. It is critical you find out before you begin how you will be paid.

Find out before you start if the client needs a copy of your insurance certificate and if there is any paperwork you need to complete in order to be paid: Many non-studio locations will require a certificate of insurance and many will require you modify it to specifically mention their site. Find all of this out before you begin, as well as if you need to fill out any other paperwork to be paid. The time to find out you needed to fill out paperwork is not after you begin teaching classes. Of course it goes without saying but you must have liability insurance to be teaching anywhere but especially when you're in a corporate setting, outside a studio.

Give both parties an "out" clause: While we never want to go into a job thinking that it won't work out, sometimes the best of intentions still do not build a successful program. Be sure that your client understands that you are there to do your best but if something unforeseen happens and/or the program is not working as expected, you reserve the right to stop teaching at any time. This rarely is a condition you'd need to invoke, but if you are in the middle of an eight class series and need to move out of the area or you're finding that the classes are not well attended, you may want to reserve the right to end the classes mid-series.

Finding and setting up these kinds of corporate yoga gigs takes a bit more time but they are great opportunities to get your name out there as an independent teacher. Once you start teaching these jobs, it's inevitable that your name will be passed along and other jobs will come your way.

Things to consider when teaching in a corporate setting

Be ready for beginners: Students in corporate classes may be unfamiliar with yoga and may be using the offer of in-office classes as a way to try it. If you only teach an all-levels or advanced sequence, streamline what you've got to the basics. I often use a six or eight class corporate series of classes to teach students alignment (as in a workshop) so that when we're done with the series, they are armed with valuable information they can take to any class they attend.

Bring mats, even if they say they have them: Even if the host says they will have mats, bring at least two. People inevitably forget them and you don't want a student to miss out, simply because they left their mat at home.

Have a sign in sheet with waiver language: In many studios, the process of signing a log or roster is also the student's signature on a release form each time they come to class. All studios have students sign an initial waiver form but many ask them to sign in again each time. When you're teaching in a corporate setting, have a manual sign in sheet and on the top of the form, have a waiver statement (see my sample form). This also serves as documentation as to how many people and who came to each class. The employer may want this information.

Focus the sequence on opening the chest, shoulders and hips: People that sit all day in front of computers will be permanently hunched forward. They'll also have a chin that juts forward, ahead of the sternum and tight hips and lower back. Present poses that open the chest, hips and shoulders and let them know why you're doing these movements and the benefit of each.

Leave the complex arm balances and headstands and handstands for your workshops: Outside of special requests, give students a general sequence that stretches, strengthens and relaxes. Along with many students who are beginners, these classes are often taught mid-day and students need to hop off their mat and back to work. Exhausting them and leaving them in a pool of sweat may not be conducive to their transition back to their desk.

Unless you can supply blocks, focus on postures that are generally accessible for students: Many students need blocks for postures like Twisting Crescent Lunge and Twisting Triangle. If you can't supply them, it doesn't hurt to offer the pose but keep in mind that what you suggest will be better appreciated if the students are grounded. I usually stay away from poses like Half Moon and Twisting Triangle because they can be frustrating without the proper support at the floor.

Understand the physical demands of their jobs and create sequencing that helps: One of my corporate wellness presentations was to an organic food delivery service. Before the meeting, I had a pre-meeting where I learned more about the various jobs in the company. Based on that, I presented poses that addressed some of the physical conditions that people might experience, given they were standing, lifting and then driving for the latter half of their day. After the presentation, a few people said their wrists and hands were tight, so I created a You Tube video they could refer to with poses specifically for the wrists and hands.

Bring layers for variable room temperatures and encourage students to do the same: I have found that in corporate settings, it's impossible to change the room temperature. As a result, sometimes it's too hot and sometimes it's too cold. As a teacher, I do not like to be cold while teaching, so I always bring an extra layer just in case. Suggest your students do the same.

Adjust the lighting but don't leave students in the dark: When you hold your corporate classes, do everything possible to avoid blasting fluorescent lights on your class. That's what they experience all day. However, don't turn the lights down so much that they are in the dark. Dark classes, except when restorative, tend to make people sleepy, so keep the lights up and if you only have fluorescent, consider turning them off and bringing in a lamp to use.

Consider leaving the chanting for the studio and explain the meaning of "Namaste": The choice of whether or not to chant before or after class and/or to say "Namaste" is up to you. In some corporate settings, you may feel like it's not a fit. Only you will be able to gauge this. However, if you do say "Namaste" after class, preface stating it with a short statement about what it means. This way, your students will know and it won't just be an automatic word they say after class.

Ask students for feedback and report this back to your business sponsor: As a point of conversation, ask students for feedback about how they feel after class. Ask them how they feel returning to their desks and in the latter part of their day. You're not asking them for feedback about the class, per se, but looking more for information about how the practice affects their bodies, minds, clarity of thinking, stress levels and attitude about their job. This is all valuable feedback for you to pass onto the business sponsor for the class, to help them see the impact the classes are making on the employees.

Special Section: Teaching to classes with mixed levels of yoga experience

One of the challenges you may face as a yoga teacher is the scenario of working a private corporate gig and having people attend with different levels of experience. This certainly can happen in a studio setting but with a privately contracted teaching job, there are other factors to consider. Things like:

- What kind of class and style of yoga were you hired to teach? A beginner's class or an all levels class?
- Is your training in Power Yoga but now that you've met the students, your sense is that something more restorative would be appropriate?
- What is the hiring contact's familiarity with yoga practice?

Privately contracted jobs give you some room to work with in terms of customizing the offering to best meet the needs of the students. In a typical studio class, the class format, style and offering is determined beforehand by the studio owner, a teacher is placed in that time slot to offer that style of yoga and for people attending, that is pretty much what they'll get (power yoga, restorative yoga, beginner's yoga, etc).

One of the scenarios that can arise in a corporate setting is that you'll find a group with mixed levels of experience (this can really happen anywhere too). Some people find that a corporate yoga offering is the perfect way to try yoga for the first time; others that have experience enjoy having class right onsite. Some companies provide incentives to employees for attending class so you may find that students who are just getting into yoga after injury or a period of inactivity also gravitate to the class. This can present some variables to you as a teacher that can be handled in a variety of ways.

Here are some tips to consider:

The best way to start any corporate teaching gig is to clarify with the sponsor the style of yoga you will be teaching. If your contact is new to yoga, you may want to have them attend one of your classes or share any DVDs or videos with them so they can get a feel for your teaching style.

Offer lots of modifications right from the start.

Share different ways to approach each posture. When you teach modifications (both to intensify and to accommodate) you educate people as to different ways to approach the pose, without having to say out loud: "And, if it's challenging to move from High to Low Push Up, drop your knees." Many people do the more intense version of Side Plank, for instance, because they have no idea they can drop their knee down. Your role is to provide many ways to do the same thing and with this approach, you allow for people with varied levels of experience to be in the same class.

Stick to a standard sequence.

It's hard for people to build competency in yoga when they're in classes with different sequences from class to class. Support your student's growth, especially at the beginning of your corporate class series, by providing the same sequence from class to class. This not only allows them to build strength, flexibility and familiarity with the flow but also allows them to build confidence and competence. This approach also allows you to be more present for them because you are less focused on what you'll offer next.

Follow up with the sponsor to discuss how the class is going.

After a few classes, if you have any thoughts about the mix of students and what you're offering and an overall concern about how the classes are going, set up a meeting with the sponsor. Bring up the issues that may be in the way of an optimal experience for everyone. If there are issues with the environment or props available, such as lack of props, noise, temperature or lighting, discuss alternate options. If you find that there are people that are regularly struggling in class, look for private times before or afterwards to ask them how they are doing. This usually will open the discussion to a point where you can offer some suggestions.

Talking to the sponsor is also a time to see if there is a potential disconnect between what you believe is needed and what he or she wants. If you find that the bulk of the class is filled with beginners but the sponsor is a hard-core practitioner who prefers a class filled with arm balances and a fast pace, talk about how you can structure a class that works for everyone.

Ask for feedback after class to see how people are doing.

As a teacher, it's easy to make assumptions about what people think of your class. The person that appears to be having an awful time may love the challenge. As people are wrapping up after class, ask them how they feel, if they have any specific questions that you can answer. This opens the door for you to offer suggestions to people who are working to build strength and familiarity with the practice.

Look for opportunities to work one on one with people who are new to yoga, working with injuries or overall lack of conditioning.

In one of my corporate classes, there were two instances where one person showed up. This student is someone who, by her own admission, is working to build strength and flexibility and is frustrated about the offerings in general yoga classes. She looks to these corporate classes as a way to get some personalized instruction. In these two instances, we worked together to create a series of modifications through the one-hour power yoga sequence so that she could feel steady and strong in each pose.

If this doesn't happen spontaneously for you with those people in your class that are having trouble, ask them if they can show up 15 or 20 minutes before class for a little individual time. This will show your investment in their time and will increase their enjoyment of the classes overall.

Suggest less effort and give examples.

Many people come to yoga with a workout mentality. The "no pain, no gain" approach to running, lifting and other gym-related workouts doesn't work as well on the mat and certainly runs against the underlying philosophy of yoga. However, many people don't know how to approach yoga poses with both strength and a sense of ease. It's your job to show them how so they can leave feeling more balanced and less stressed. Things like holding poses and encouraging breath, speaking to the parts of the body that should be relaxing as other parts work, the use of props, the use of resting in Child's Pose if one feels pushed to an edge; these are all tools that people can use to help them manage their energy and effort in class.

Closing Summary

Your role as a teacher in these corporate settings is as the expert. You're not only providing the classes but any background information on the benefits of yoga as a practice. In a corporate setting, it is helpful to mention how yoga can increase your ability to be focused, clear and less reactive. Also remind people of how the poses they do to stretch hips and shoulders are great to do during the day, to stretch out a body that is tight from sitting. Be confident and clear in your approach and look for ways to accommodate everyone. You'll be making a contribution to their yoga practice and giving the students tools they can use as they take class in studio or on their own as well as tools to help them improve the health of their job.

Chapter 23

Teaching Students with Injuries and Specific Medical Conditions

Focus

This chapter will provide techniques for teaching yoga to individuals with a variety of medical conditions and injuries, as well as those with overall physical conditioning that may require customized modifications. These students may require a bit more customization but there is always a way to create a sequence that works for each person.

Overall Considerations

The practice of yoga can be modified for just about anyone, with any medical condition, injury or in any particular physical condition. The mindset of the yoga teacher needs to be focused on the essentials of a healthy yoga practice: breathing, connecting to the foundation of the body (i.e., whatever is at the floor) and staying present. The mindset of the yoga teacher should not be focused on the idea of "perfect poses," "correcting students" and the idea of "wrong or right."

The ability to highly customize a practice for a particular individual varies when working with a student in a group class in a studio or other setting versus working with a student privately. Here are some factors to consider for both settings:

- When working with group class, it is not always known what conditions individuals have, unless their condition is able to be determined by looking at them or they tell you before class begins. As a result, you may be in the middle of class and realize through observation that a student is struggling or attempting to modify.

- Depending on the size of the class, it may or may not be possible for you to 1- get to that student to provide hands-on assistance 2- talk quietly with the student about what's going on, while holding the other students in a pose 3- know definitively what the student's condition is from observation only. As a result, you may need to manage the situation as it is happening.

- As you watch the student struggle, especially if you can't get to them in that moment, you may have feelings of pity or frustration. You may feel sorry for the person. You may even feel some anger that they selected your class and did not share with you before the class their personal situation. It is important to let these feeling go and stay present. It is not your job to rescue the student. In fact, part of the practice is for the student (within reason) to tap into their sense of what would work best for them and act on it.

- Make sure you have props quickly available to you as the teacher. Students may not take blocks or straps and if reaching them quickly to provide to a student in need is hard for you, given where they are stored, grab a few before class and have them nearby. Also, you may want to make a general statement before each class about taking props. However, many students will not know what props they need and especially won't know the right block size to use and how many blocks to use for many of the customized modifications that might be appropriate (such as using blocks under the hands for someone with wrist pain). Therefore, you have to think ahead and have them nearby so you can get to them quickly.

- If a student gets up to leave, it may or may not be possible to talk to them before they leave the room. If you have a way to put the class in pose and connect with the student, do so. Ask them, "Is there a way I can help?" Always lead with compassion, never with, "What's wrong? Why did you leave?" You can only assume it's related to their physical challenges but you will not be sure until you speak to them directly. If you can't get to them, other than making sure they are physically safe to leave (which will most likely be the case if they walked out on their own), there is nothing you can do. Make a mental note and try to connect with them the next time you see them (if you do, which of course, you hope you do).

- If you are able to get to them, encourage them to come back, even if it's just to rest on the floor. Or, if you are in the standing series, encourage them to come back for floor work and then shavasana.

- It is up to you if you wish to ask students before class if anyone has a condition or injury they wish to share. This really depends on the teacher, his or her comfort level with managing the responses one might receive and keeping the class moving forward. Also, most students may not share in a group setting even when asked so it is highly unlikely you will get the information you need.

- If you have a student that approaches you before class to share the details of a particular condition, take the time to be sure their mat is placed in a location conducive for you to reach them during class and also one that affords them a little privacy. Putting a student like this in the front row (which is where they may place themselves if they walk into the room and get overwhelmed with where to go) will be distracting to the other students and possibly make the student feel self-conscious. The point is not to hide the student but to have them somewhere in the room where they have space for props, you can see them clearly and can reach them. The way this is handled can be a bit of a challenge, especially if you have a full class and need to ask an existing student from the back or middle row to move to the front. More discussion may be needed on this topic but know that as long as you lead with compassion and stay neutral to any angry feedback you get, you will be moving in the right direction. If the bottom line is you cannot put the student where you'd like, know that it is fine, and you and he/she will do the best with what is available.

- When working with a student privately, before meeting for the first time, gather general information about the student's goals for yoga and ask general questions about any injuries or medical conditions. The first session will be devoted to gathering more information, but be prepared by having asked before your first session. Also, just because a student says they have a specific condition, does not mean they will exhibit symptoms and functional challenges according to general guidelines. It is always necessary to have this information in the background and then see how the student's body is upon the first meeting.

Remember that in all instances, if you are asked a question by a student with a certain condition and don't know the answer, say, "I don't know but I will get back to you." Use it as an opportunity to learn something new and find out how to reach the student so you can get back to them or tell them you will let them know when they come back to class on (set a specific date).

Remember that your job is not to treat any condition medically. Unless you are a physician as well as a yoga teacher (and even in that case, you are not formally treating the student in your capacity as a physician) it is inappropriate for you to give out medical advice around taking medications or even holistic remedies. It is generally appropriate for you to make suggestions, or speak from personal experience (i.e., "What I have found works for my migraines is…..") but it is not within your purview as a teacher to suggest specific treatment.

It is very rare that someone will have a medical emergency in your class or private. However, as a general rule for all classes and privates, have a phone nearby. Be sure you are first aid and CPR certified. In an emergency, your first job is to check the student and stay with him/her and identify a specific person who will call 911 and report back to you that they have been called. You do NOT leave the student to call 911; you stay with him/her. Also, do not make a general statement to "call 911!" Make sure you delegate quickly and specifically so you know they have been called. Stay with the student until medical help arrives. Provide your contact information to the rescue personnel so they can reach you for details if necessary and also so that the family members can contact you, if need be.

If you have a student that needs assistance and he or she refuses your offer of a prop or a modification, move on. This might be in the context of a group class or even a private session. Try not to take it personally and stay neutral.

General Modifications, their Application and working with Specific Conditions

Your primary role as a teacher in working with people with different kinds of physical challenges is to make the practice accessible for them without talking down to them or babying them. Treating the student with respect and avoiding pity will go a long way in developing a relationship based on mutual respect.

There is much you can learn from the student about their medical condition and much of what you apply to their practice can be re-purposed with other students (to a certain extent) so it is very valuable to you as a teacher to work with people of all physical abilities. This also gives you a way to increase your marketability as a teacher; through your exposure to students of different ages, body types and physical capability levels, you will gain experience you can use to pursue teaching jobs in nursing homes, hospitals, senior living centers, rehabilitation centers as well as non-profits and organizations that support individuals with certain medical conditions. It will also make you a stronger teacher because you'll be able to manage anyone that comes to your classes. It will also help you develop a deep appreciation for the practice of yoga and it's applicability to all body types, ages and ability levels.

Many of these tips will work best in a private setting although some may work in a group setting if you have time to provide the modification to the student:

Finding a comfortable seat: In order to work with a student with any kind of medical condition, disability or physical challenge due to age, weight or other condition, it is helpful to find a seated position from which you can begin to work. This grounds the student and gives you a place to start them breathing without the added complication or challenge that standing or holding a pose can bring. Seated options can include a chair, a block, a block and blanket and could involve sitting in Easy pose, Hero's pose or even a Straddle. A block may be needed or a chair to provide a solid foundation from which to provide support. If necessary, sitting a student against a flat wall is helpful as well.

Connecting Breathing and Movement: Once the student is seated in a customized way, you can begin with simple movements and address the breath. Breathing in on upward movements and breathing out on downward movements can begin to provide the student with an awareness of how deep breathing feels in the body, can start to trigger the relaxation response and can begin to give you an idea of their coordination, strength, proprioception (sense of their limbs in space) and ability to follow verbal directions. It also gives you both a chance to start to assess the impact that movement has on the body. Ask the student for feedback during these initial movements with open-ended questions such as, "How does that feel?" Keep them open-ended so as not to lead the student in any particular way.

Child's Pose: A great pose to insert early on is Child's Pose. Not only will it stretch the spine and open the hips, it's a powerful pose in that it brings the student into their breath and shifts them from distraction to connection.
*Students with knee problems, use a blanket under the knees.
*Students with tight hips, place a blanket or block between hips and heels.

Introducing twisting movements: Once you have moved through some initial movements from seated, you can add simple twists from the seat as well. Bringing a hand to the opposite knee, instructing the student to ground down into the hips (hence the reason for the solid seat) and turn their torso towards the hand on the knee can provide a basic twisting motion. This will allow them to work the mid- to upper back, which typically is very tight in most people. Again, ask for feedback throughout to assess how the student is doing and to make further modifications as needed.

Moving to basic poses close to the floor: Once you have moved through these sequences, paying close attention to the breath and getting feedback from the student, introduce some basic poses. Two of the best ones to start with are Tabletop and Downward Facing Dog. Tabletop is less strenuous than Downward Dog but can provide you with a chance to speak to "stacking the joints," a critical piece of alignment and also can give you a chance to lead the student through a series of Cat/Cow movements, which again will allow them to breathe and move together.
*If they are uncomfortable on their knees, a blanket underneath can provide relief.

Be sure to provide lots of support around bending the knees in Downward Dog and explain the basic function of the pose is to stretch the spine. Speak to alignment (feet hip width, hands shoulder width).

* If they are uncomfortable on their hands, you can place them on two blocks of equal size.
*If they start with labored breathing, only hold Downward Dog for 3 breaths, rest, and then try again.

*Certain medical conditions may preclude a student having their head lower than their heart. This could include migraines, glaucoma and high blood pressure. If so, avoid the pose completely.

Backbending, including Cobra and Upward Facing Dog: As much as Downward Facing Dog is strenuous for many students, Upward Facing Dog can be just as challenging. The movement requires upper body strength as well as lower body awareness, as well as spinal flexibility. Most people have good mobility in their lower back but not their mid or upper back so the full bending of the back is difficult.

To start, get the student lying on the floor: Have them bring their arms by their sides, like Airplane Pose, but on the belly. On an inhale, have them lift their chest, drop their chin, extend back through the legs and take 3 breaths. Use this as a chance to evaluate their spinal flexibility as well as their ability to integrate their legs into the pose.

From there, move into Cobra pose. Cobra will give them a chance to bring more effort into the pose because they are pressing into their hands. Have them come up to low Cobra and take a few breaths, noticing the same thing as in the earlier pose.

From there, if all is going well and they are not struggling, bring them into full Upward Facing Dog. Be sure to notice if the shoulders are up by the ears and if so, have them drop them down the back.

* If they are uncomfortable on their hands, (which could be from any repetitive stress injury like carpal tunnel or just general de-conditioning) have them use blocks of equal size under each hand. This will raise them off the floor and also take some of the pressure off the hands. In some bodies this makes no difference and they still complain of wrist pain. If so, drop them down in intensity to one of the other modifications/poses.
* Students that have had a spinal fusion in any part of the spine will have trouble extending (bending) their back. For these students, it is critical they bring leg strength into the pose but they may also need to work a low Cobra pose for now or forever. It is up to you to help them realize that this is fine. However, they may see slow changes over time that allows them to extend their spine further. For these students, it is also very helpful to be on blocks because that lifts them off the floor a

bit higher, which may help them get into a fuller backbend.

Standing Poses: Bringing the student to his/her feet and working basic poses, such as Tadasana, Warrior 1, Warrior Two, Chair Pose and Triangle will allow them to move more and give you a chance to assess their ability further. Be sure to have blocks available for Triangle, use a wider, shorter stance for Warrior Poses if need be and separate the feet to hip width in Chair if it is more comfortable.

Connecting Standing Poses to Floor Poses/ Moving into Vinyasa/ Sun Salutations: Two of the most basic sequences in yoga are Sun Salutation A and Sun Salutation B. If you can leave a student with an understanding of how to move through these two sequences, you will have given them a way to integrate yoga into their day easily, as even just 10 minutes of these basic movements can connect them to their breath and body. However, for many students, it is difficult to move from Downward Dog to Warrior 1; they don't have the strength and flexibility to step forward. So, a modification is needed.

From standing, have the student bow forward and move through half-way lift into Plank. As needed, have them drop the knees to lower to Low Push Up. If this movement is too challenging, avoid it all together and simply have them move from Plank to Downward Dog.

• Students with lower back issues, such as fusions or herniated discs may not be able to tolerate forward folds. Skip them all together and have them drop to their hands and knees to enter Downward Dog.

From Downward Dog, have them step their right foot forward and use their hand to bring their foot under the knee. From there, have them press up to Warrior 1. If this is too challenging, have them step forward to a lunge, with the back knee down, reach up and then lift the back knee. If it is still too challenging, avoid lifting the knee all together and keep the knee down. In that case, have them do Warrior 1 as a stand-alone pose only entered from standing.

Once you have moved through some Sun Salutations in whatever modified way is necessary, you can add in Warrior Two and Triangle and begin to move the student through a vinyasa practice for as long as appropriate.

Balancing Poses: Balancing poses are an excellent way for students to connect to their feet, create a sense of "balance" in their body and from that, they can often evoke feelings of strength, peace, calm and confidence. For many students, balance will be tough. They have not tried it before or ever, nothing else in their functional day to day movements require that they balance on one foot and their ankles may be weak. It may be very disorienting for them to stand on one foot and feelings of frustration may come up.

Basic balancing poses like Tree and Airplane are challenging enough to allow the student to develop the skill of balancing on one foot and also provide lots of opportunities for modification. For Tree Pose, the foot on the opposite leg can be close to the ground or touching; for Airplane, the back foot can be down on the floor. As the student gets more confident and experienced, he/she can lift the leg higher in either pose. * For the student experiencing vertigo or any condition that leads to dizziness, have them modify by dropping the foot in either pose or holding onto a chair.

Backbends/ Hips: Once you are through with balancing, bring the student to their backs. Bridge Pose is an excellent entry-level backbend and very effective in stretching the hip flexors. You can place a block under the student for support, especially if they can't tolerate holding the pose.

*For students with vertigo or other neck conditions, it may be uncomfortable for them to be lying on their back. If this is the case, do not put something under the head; avoid the pose all together.

If the student wants to try Upward Bow Pose, commonly called Wheel, support them with blocks under their hands and coming to the crown of their head to start (only do this if they can be up against a wall). For students with very stiff spines, they will be in more of a "flat back/upside down" versus an "arched" back. For these students, it is important to help them gain flexibility in the mid- and upper spine and the earlier floor work with Cobra and Upward Dog, over time, will help with this. Be sure to reinforce "bringing the elbows in" which will allow for more space in the back.

Pigeon: Offer the student the chance to do this pose the traditional way, lying face down on the floor but also give them the modified version where they are lying on their back if necessary. Use ample props, like a blanket under the hip and a block under the head to bring the spine into a more neutral position and the cervical spine into less flexion.

Shavasana: To set the student up, have them lay on their back. If this is uncomfortable for any reason, have them lay on their right side (unless pregnant, then it's the left side). Use props such as a blanket over the hips. Do not put anything under the head. Have them open their hands towards the ceiling (unless they are on their side). Leave them for 5 minutes minimum. If they want, cover their eyes with a towel.

Additional Tips

Students with glaucoma, blood pressure problems or vertigo may not tolerate having the head lower than the heart. Avoid poses that put them in this position.

Students with shoulder concerns, such as rotator cuff injuries, will only aggravate their condition by moving from High to Low Push up, then Upward Dog and to Downward Dog. Have them simply move from High Push Up directly into Downward Dog.

Students that are not yet strong enough to at least safely be on the crown of the head in Wheel should do Bridge or Supported Bridge.

Many poses can be modified for a person sitting in a chair. This might be appropriate for an elderly person or someone who uses a wheelchair.

Students with repetitive wrist injuries, such as carpel tunnel, should use blocks under the hands to decrease the angle of the wrist in Downward Dog. Also, "Grip Its" (a yoga prop that looks like small dumbbells you place under each hand) can be used instead of blocks or flat hands.

Closing Summary

Overall, keep in mind that your job is to lead with compassion and be a guide for the student, helping them find their breath, connect to their body and also, help them have some compassion for their body as well. By the same token, encourage them, set reasonable goals and maintain as regular a schedule as possible, emphasizing that it's not so much " how long" you practice or but more that you do even just a little bit, every day.

Weekly Worksheet of Activities

WEEK OF: Sunday _____ thru Saturday_____

Sample Business Tasks:
Update Linked In Profile
Make one new contact

Billing:
Studio A Monthly Submit
Studio B Weekly Submit

Personal Practice:
Book 2 yoga classes per week

Marketing:
Update Website
Daily Facebook posts
Daily Twitter posts

Writing:
Blog post
Article A
Article B

Weekly Business Documents:
Complete weekly report
Update business leads
Update revenue figures
Enter all classes on teaching log

Data:
Back up computer
Synch Phone

Bills
Bill A by X date
Bill B by Y date

Transfers
Transfer amount to personal savings
Transfer amount to business savings for taxes

Weekly Business Report

Week Ending:
Date:

Summary of Weekly Activity (by date):

Yoga classes taught:

New Contacts Made:
New Closed Deals (Entity/Service/Revenue):
Lost deals:

Weekly Revenue Generated (Service/Revenue/ Method of Payment):

--insert spreadsheet section

Total: $

Business Expenses:

--insert spreadsheet section

Total: $

Next week's planned activities:

Completed Tasks this week:

Monthly Revenue Projection for Month of January as of this reporting period:
Monthly Revenue Surplus or Shortfall:

Overall Assessment of Week:

Jane Doe

Street Address
City, State Zip Code
555-555-5555
jane@email.com
www.website.com

Highlights

- General statement about non-yoga work experience
- Statement that illustrates why you teach yoga and what makes you unique
- Transition statement that illustrates why you have decided to focus on teaching yoga (versus continue to work in your field of initial training)

Teaching Background

- Designation through Yoga Alliance (if any)
- Certifications (if any)
- Style of yoga taught
- Years of experience teaching
- Significant trainings attended
- Specialties (children, seniors, athletes, privates, chronic pain, etc)

(Include all work experience, both in yoga industry and in general corporate industry)
(List studios and any other location where you teach yoga)

Employer, City, State
Start date-End date
Job title
- Action and result oriented responsibility
- Action and result oriented responsibility
- Action and result oriented responsibility

Employer, City, State
Start date-End date
Job Title
- Action and result oriented responsibility
- Action and result oriented responsibility
- Action and result oriented responsibility

Employer, City, State
Start date-End date
Job Title
- Action and result oriented responsibility

- Action and result oriented responsibility
- Action and result oriented responsibility

Employer, City, State
Start date-End date
Job Title
- Action and result oriented responsibility
- Action and result oriented responsibility

Education

School name, City, State	Dates attended
Degree awarded	
School name, City, State	Dates attended
Degree awarded	

Other Highlights
Include significant achievements that may have a bearing on your teaching and experience
Volunteer experience if relevant
Related passions if relevant

Business Expenses Sample Tracking Worksheet

Date	Item	Location/Vendor	Cost	Method of payment	Category
1/1/14	Office Supplies	Staples	$12.00	Bank A Debit Card	Office Supplies

Sample Teaching Log

Date	Location	Rate (gross)	Paid?	Tax status	Hours	No. of Students	Time	Notes	Dollar amount taxes
1/1/14	Boston Yoga	$50	no	no	1	20	6:30am		$10.00

Sample Budget Log

Rent or Mortgage
Condo fee if applicable
Utility
Utility

Home internet and cable provider
Email provider
Mobile Phone

Credit card payments
Any loan payments

Car Insurance
Gasoline costs
Any monthly parking fees
Homeowner's insurance
Health Insurance
Any other monthly medical costs

Weekly spending money for all
miscellaneous expenses

Estimated tax payment to IRS
Estimated tax payment to State
Personal Savings (cash)
Personal Savings (IRA)
Total:

Business Dashboard Sample

Dream Big Number (Desired annual gross salary)	$50,000.00			
Monthly Target	$4,166.00			
Weekly Target	$1,041.00			
Daily Target (6D / week)	$173.50			

Activities*	Rate per Activity	Classes per week	Total revenue per week	Comments
Items in black are existing classes				
Items in red are yet to be booked (marketing opportunities)				
Items in blue are booked but have not started yet				
Studio classes				
Studio A	$50.00	2	$100.00	
Studio B	$60.00	3	$180.00	
Studio C	$50.00	2	$100.00	
Studio D	$50.00	1	$50.00	
Studio E	$50.00	1	$50.00	
Total studio teaching	**$480/week**		**$1920/month**	
Corporate Yoga				
Corporation A	$75.00	1	$75.00	
Corporation B	$100.00	1	$100.00	
Corporation C	$100.00	1	$100.00	
Corporation D	$100.00	1	$100.00	
Total corporate teaching	**$375/week**		**$1500/month**	
Privates				
Client A	$100.00	1	$100.00	
Client B	$100.00	2	$200.00	
Total private client teaching	**$300/week**		**$1200/month**	
Workshops				
Training 1	$100.00	1	$100/month	
Training 2	$100.00	1	$100/month	
Total workshop/training teaching			**$200/month**	
Total revenue teaching			$4820/month	
Total overage for plan			$654	
Unbooked revenue included in above calculation			$1200/month	
Actual revenue at present			$3620/month	
Total shortage at present			($566/month)	

* refers to using color coding

Sample Statement Of Work Form

Thank you for contacting me regarding yoga services and programs. The following document outlines the services that we have agreed to and the terms of the service.

Once you have reviewed this, please send a hard copy back with your signature. A hard copy will be sent to you with a self-addressed stamped envelope to make it easy to return.

Thank you!

Client:

Address:

Telephone Number:

Email address:

Service Requested:

Dates of Services:

Rate for service:

Payment Terms (form of payment, frequency of payment):

Special conditions (if any):

Any special notes:

Supplies/ Equipment and who will provide:

Liability Insurance document requested:

Any special paperwork that needs to be completed prior to job:

General Terms of Service:
- Indicate if mats will be brought by you or supplied by client
- Indicate cancelation procedures if a class needs to be canceled
- Either party can terminate this agreement at any time without penalty
- Other

Contact Information:

Your mailing address

Your email address

Your telephone number

Your website

Signed:

(Your name)

Signed:

(Your client's signature)

Sample Release Form**

I understand and agree to the following:

1. I am participating in yoga classes during which I will receive information and instruction about yoga and health. I recognize that yoga requires physical exertion, which may be strenuous and may cause physical injury and I am fully aware of the risks and hazards involved.
2. I understand that it is my responsibility to consult with a physician prior to and regarding my participation in yoga classes. I represent and warrant that I am physically fit and have no medical condition that would prevent my full participation in yoga classes.
3. I agree to assume full responsibility for any risks, injuries or damages, known or unknown, which I might incur as a result of participating in yoga classes.
4. I knowingly and expressly waive any claim I may have against XXXXX for injury or damages that I may sustain as a result of participating in yoga classes.

I have read the above release and waiver of liability and fully understand its contents. I voluntarily agree to the terms and conditions stated above.

Name (Print):

Name (Sign):

** This is only a sample and should be considered only a suggested format

Closing Remarks

Teaching yoga is a rewarding career that can be done full time or on the side. For that reason alone, it's a completely versatile career that can change as your life circumstances shift. Regardless of the model you use, it's always your passion for sharing this timeless tradition that will fuel you through days you love to teach and days you feel awkward and closed off. Your expression of teaching will change as you do and as you develop more skill and experience, you'll worry less about what you say and develop more confidence and comfort around just being yourself.

Even the newest teachers can bring the most important skill that one needs to teach yoga: the quality of being yourself. I wish you all the best as you pursue this wonderfully rewarding path.

Namaste.

Acknowledgements

There are so many people that I wish to thank for helping me create this book. First of all, thank you to my parents who have supported me through the journey of my teaching career so far, including the development of this book. Thanks to my brother, Mark, who is an amazing writer and had wonderful feedback to share with me about writing this book. Thank you to my sweetie, Ben Reese, for being a tireless support and listener about the "stretching" my yoga career has taken me through so far. You have always been there for me. Special thanks to my dear friends, Bruce Blake and Cedric Adams, my unofficial "Board of Directors," for your ongoing guidance over the years as well as to the content and planning for this book. Thanks to author and friend Andrew Davis, for lending your wonderful insight to the development of this project as well as Debra Ball, my dear friend with a most amazing eye for visuals, layouts and the printed word. Thanks to the test readers that lent me their time in reading the book draft and provided me with wonderful, insightful feedback. Thank you to Kristin Quinn, owner of Charlestown Yoga, for connecting me to the fabulous Alessandra Tortorello, who worked to create the format for submission to Create Space. This project would never have been completed without all of you. I am forever grateful.

Karen Fabian
April 2, 2014
Boston, MA

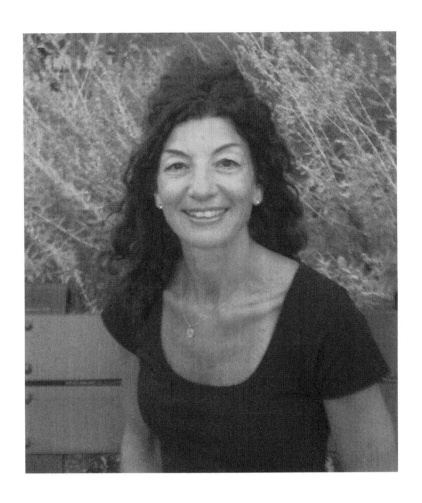

About the Author

Karen Fabian has been teaching yoga since 2002. She is the Founder of Bare Bones Yoga, her yoga business devoted to "keeping yoga simple." This motto reflects her passion for providing students with the essentials to increase strength and flexibility. She's registered with Yoga Alliance as an Experienced Registered Teacher and is a Certified Baptiste Yoga Teacher. She is currently completing an advanced 500 Hour training program with teacher Tiffany Cruikshank.

Karen teaches studio-based classes, meets with clients individually and has been teaching children in a variety of settings for over 10 years. She works with crew teams and individual rowers in a variety of training centers and leads corporate classes in businesses in Boston. She has a mentorship program for teachers, gives presentations on wellness topics to businesses in Boston and teaches anatomy to yoga teachers.

She is a regular contributor to online yoga publications, including MindBodyGreen, YOGANONOMOUS.com and DoYouYoga.com.

Karen's academic background is in Physical therapy and Rehabilitation Counseling and she has her Bachelor's Degree from Boston University. She also has a Master's in Health Care Administration from Simmons College. She has over 20 years of corporate business experience working in healthcare and software development. She lives in Boston with her loveable yellow lab, Bailey Rose.

Her website is www.barebonesyoga.com. She can be reached via email at karen@barebonesyoga.com.

This content is proprietary to Bare Bones Yoga and Karen Fabian. Any unauthorized use, distribution or copying of this document is restricted.

For further information, see www.barebonesyoga.com

Made in the USA
Charleston, SC
03 September 2014